Myasthenia Gravis

An Illustrated History

John Carl Keesey, M.D.

Publishers Design Group
Roseville, California

Library of Congress Control Number: 2001097858

Book and cover design: Robert Brekke

ISBN: 1-929170-04-1

Publishers Design Group
Roseville, CA 95678
www.publishersdesign.com
800.587.6666

Printed in China

Contents

Acknowledgments

THIS BOOK WOULD NOT EXIST WERE IT NOT FOR THE ENCOURAGEMENT and persistence of Lois Pedersen, M.S., Executive Director of the Myasthenia Gravis Foundation of California, who raised the funds to make it possible, found translators for the old German articles, obtained permissions for illustrations, and shepherded the numerous revisions through the design and review processes. Those fighting the battle against MG are lucky to have Lois in their corner, and I very much wish to acknowledge and thank her for all her valuable help!

A generous gift from Jack and Jean Craemer to the Myasthenia Gravis Foundation of California was the stimulus that made this book possible in the first place. The Craemers have been very supportive of the activities of the Myasthenia Gravis Foundation of California, and I appreciate their generosity.

Interested as I am in the history of medicine, I feel disadvantaged by my inability to read German. I am therefore very grateful for the conscientious efforts of the volunteer translators of the three seminal articles in difficult old medical German which are featured in Chapter 1: For Erb's 1879 paper, Dr. Stephen M. Coutts, Executive Vice-President of Research & Development for La Jolla Pharmaceutical Company; for Goldflam's 1893 paper, Ms. Karin Molnar of the California Hospital Medical Center; and for Jolly's 1895 paper, Mr. Ron Hay. I hope that the complete English translations of these important papers, now that they are available, will find a permanent home on an MG history website someday. I wish also to thank Martina Wiedau-Pazos, M.D., Ph.D., for facile *ad hoc* German translations as needed.

Karen Hudson, Mathilda Karel Spak, Luis Chui, M.D., Daniel Drachman, M.D., David Grob, M.D., Donald Mulder, M.D., Arthur Strauss, M.D., and Frisca Yan-Go, M.D., each helped me at specific times during the preparation of the posters or of this book, and to each of them I extend my sincere thanks. And I am particularly grateful to Johan Aarli, M.D., Andrew Engel, M.D., David Richman, M.D., and Stanley Way, who reviewed the entire manuscript and made this book better by their suggestions. Of course, any errors of fact or judgment are mine alone.

—JOHN KEESEY, M.D.
Pacific Palisades, California
September 24, 2001

Preface

SEVERAL YEARS BEFORE THE CONDITION which came to be known as Myasthenia Gravis had even been recognized, the great French neurologist Jean Martin Charcot remarked in 1857 that "Disease is very old, and nothing about it has changed. It is we who change, as we learn to recognize what was formerly imperceptible."

The truth of this statement becomes apparent as one traces the gradual evolution of our understanding of what we now call "MG", an uncommon but challenging disease characterized by fluctuating fatigue and weakness of skeletal muscles, including eye muscles, limb muscles, and those muscles used for chewing, swallowing, talking, and breathing. During the past twenty five years, while I have cared for many patients with MG, I have been a witness to the burgeoning information which makes up the latter part of this story. But the earlier history of MG is interesting as well, a time when physicians tried to define and understand a fluctuating condition which often seemed to have no observable pathology.

In 1997, during the Ninth International Conference on Myasthenia Gravis and Related Disorders in Santa Monica, California, I attempted to illustrate the highlights of our changing perceptions about MG over the past one hundred years on a series of four-foot-square posters. I was supported in this endeavor by Lois Pedersen, M.S., Executive Director of the Myasthenia Gravis Foundation of California, with inspired artistic assistance from Alexandra Manley, B.F.A., and her assistant, my son Patrick Keesey, B.F.A. Reaction of the myasthenia experts at the Conference towards the content of the posters was generally favorable, and some of them expressed the hope that eventually this illustrated history could find a more accessible home. The recent opportunity to transform the posters into a book was made possible by a generous gift to the Myasthenia Gravis Foundation of California from Jack and Jean Craemer of San Rafael, California, to whom I wish to express my special gratitude.

A glossary of technical terms used in this book has been added to assist non-medical readers.

Clinical Recognition (1879-1901)

Introduction

Few specific neurological disease entities had been delineated when in the middle of the 19th century the French neurologist Jean Martin Charcot and his associates in Paris began "to extract a specific pathological state from the chaos of imprecision," as he was quoted as saying. His method emphasized precision of clinical observation and exactitude of anatomical analysis.

One of the earliest successes of this approach was the 1860 description by Charcot's colleague, Duchenne de Bologne, of progressive weakness of the tongue, lips, and soft palate ("la paralysie glosso-labiolaryngée") which soon came to be known in English as "progressive bulbar palsy." The "bulb" was an early term for the brainstem, that portion of the central nervous system between the cerebral cortex or "brain" and the spinal cord beginning in the neck. The cell bodies of nerves supplying the muscles of the face, tongue, and throat originate in the brainstem or "bulb," and Duchenne postulated that the characteristic wasting (atrophy) of the tongue in this condition was caused by degeneration of the nerve cells in the brainstem.

Compared to the steady downhill course of progressive bulbar palsy, some patients had a fluctuating and even remitting course of muscle weakness made worse by use of those muscles and improved with rest. Three papers in German during the last quarter of the Nineteenth Century established that this condition was different from the progressive bulbar palsy of Duchenne.

Wilhelm Erb, 1879

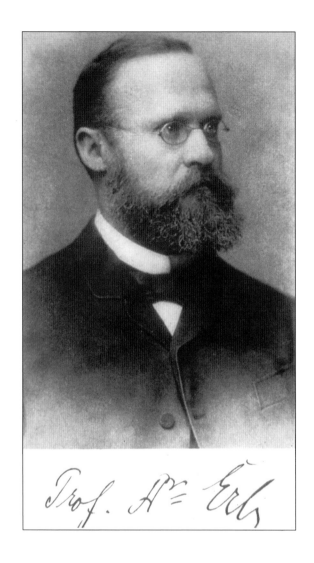

Wilhelm Heinrich Erb was the first person to suggest that there might be a unique form of bulbar palsy which did not follow the inexorable downhill course of typical progressive bulbar palsy.

In 1878 he presented a three-part paper on the bulbar palsies at a meeting of neurologists and psychiatrists in Germany which was published in 1879 in the medical journal *Archiv für Psychiatrie und Nervenkrankheiten*[1]. In the third part of this paper he described "Einen neuen, wahrscheinlich bulbären Symptomencomplex" (A new probably bulbar symptom-complex) in three patients whom he had seen in 1868, 1870, and 1871. (He was not to meet another similar case for twenty years.)

The features which he thought differentiated this new condition from progressive bulbar palsy were bilateral drooping eyelids ("ptosis"), severe neck weakness (neck "paresis"), and trouble chewing.

Two of Erb's patients actually made apparent recoveries during the short time Erb followed them before writing his paper, but the third patient, a 30-year-old woman, died suddenly in the night after one and one-half years of remissions and relapses. No autopsy was performed, but Erb presumed that the origin of the disease was in the brainstem.

Erb was 38 years old when this paper was published, and if not already the leading neurologist in Germany, he would soon be considered such. Samuel Goldflam compared Erb's cases to his own three cases fourteen years later.

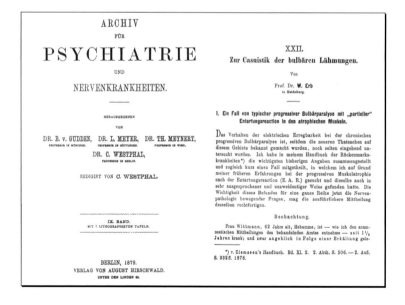

Below on the left is a table from Erb's paper in which he compares the clinical features of each of his patients. An English translation of the table appears on the right. Erb stated that *"Each of these case histories contains certain related symptoms, many of which are uncommon. Although I do not intend to suggest that these three cases document the same pathologic-anatomical illness, said symptoms do confirm my premise that the site of pathological occurrences is the same or very similar among them. I have constructed the following tables in the interest of emphasizing the parallels which exist among the three cases I have discussed. Although different with regard to the order of their appearance and the degree of their severity, the symptoms charted in the following table reflect significant congruencies among the three cases."*

Fall 1.	Fall 2.	Fall 3.
Entwicklung unter Kopf- und Nackenschmerzen in einigen Monaten.	Entwicklung unter Kopfweh und Schwindel, leichten Gesichtszuckungen, Doppelsehen in einigen Monaten.	Entwicklung unter Kopfschmerzen, Schwindel, Schwäche der Extremitäten in einigen Monaten.
Ptosis. Parese der Nackenmuskeln. Atrophie derselben.	Ptosis. Schwäche d. Nackenmuskeln.	Ptosis. Schwäche d. Nackenmuskeln.

344   Prof. Dr. W. Erb,

Fall 1.	Fall 2.	Fall 3.
Parese der Kaumuskeln. Atrophie derselben.	Parese der Kaumuskeln. Oefter Zuckungen derselben.	Schwäche der Kaumuskeln.
Zunge schwerbeweglich.	Zunge zitternd, später mager.	Zunge etw. schwach.
Erschwerung d. Schlingens.	Erschwerung des Schlingens.	Schlingen gut.
Oberes Facialisgebiet: normal.	Oberes Facialisgebiet: leichte Reizung (klonische Zuckungen.)	Oberes Facialisgebiet: leichte Parese mit Reizungserscheinungen.
Unteres Facialisgebiet: normal.	Unteres Facialisgebiet: normal.	Unteres Facialisgebiet: normal.
Augenbewegungen: normal.	Augenbewegungen: alle sehr mangelhaft.	Augenbewegungen: normal.
Ohrensausen. Hyperästhes. Nerv. acust. sin.	Ohrensausen; anomale Reaction des Acustic. sin.	—
—	Vermehrter Speichelfluss.	—
Leichte Schwäche der Arme.	Grosse Schwäche der Extremitäten.	Grosse Schwäche der Extremitäten.

Case 1	Case 2	Case 3
• Development of headaches, neck pain and dizziness within several months	• Development of headaches, dizziness, mild facial spasms and double vision within several months	• Development of headaches, neck pain, and weakness of the limbs within several months
• Ptosis	• Ptosis	• Ptosis
• Paralysis and atrophy of neck muscles	• Weakness of the neck muscles	• Weakness of the neck muscles
• Paralysis and atrophy of masticatory muscles	• Paralysis and frequent spasms of the masticatory muscles	• Weakness of the masticatory muscles
• Difficulty in moving tongue	•Tongue involuntarily mobile; later thin	• Tongue slightly weak
• Difficulty in swallowing	• Difficulty in swallowing	• Swallowing normal
• Upper facial area normal	• Upper facial area subject to minor irritation (chronic spasms)	• Upper facial area afflicted with mild paralysis and irritation
• Lower facial area normal	• Lower facial area normal	• Lower facial area normal
• Eye movements normal	• Eye movements all significantly impaired	• Eye movements normal
• Buzzing in the ears; auditory nerve deficit	• Buzzing in the ears; abnormal auditory reaction	
	• Increased flow of saliva	
• Slight weakness of the arms	• Severe weakness of the extremities	• Severe weakness of the extremities

(English translations by Stephen M. Coutts, Ph.D., with permission)

Samuel Goldflam, 1893

Samuel Goldflam was a physician in Warsaw, Poland, who had established out of his own earnings a polyclinic for poor patients with neurological disorders.

Because all three of the patients whom Goldflam described were in remission or much improved at the time of his paper, he entitled it "Ueber einen scheinbar heilbaren bulbärparalytischen Symptomencomplex mit Betheiligung der Extremitäten"[2] (About an apparently curable bulbar paralytic symptom-complex with involvement of the extremities).

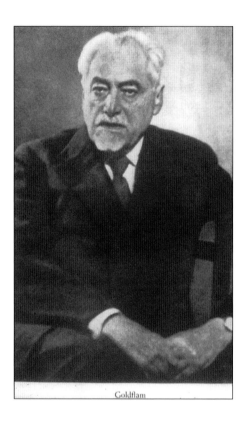

Goldflam

DEUTSCHE ZEITSCHRIFT

FÜR

NERVENHEILKUNDE.

HERAUSGEGEBEN

VON

Prof. Wilh. Erb.
Director der med. Klinik in Heidelberg.

Prof. L. Lichtheim.
Director der med. Klinik in Königsberg.

Prof. Fr. Schultze.
Director der med. Klinik in Bonn.

Prof. Ad. Strümpell.
Director der med. Klinik in Erlangen.

DRITTER BAND.

Mit 37 Abbildungen im Text und 7 Tafeln.

LEIPZIG,
VERLAG VON F. C. W. VOGEL.
1893.

XVII.

Ueber einen scheinbar heilbaren bulbärparalytischen Symptomencomplex mit Betheiligung der Extremitäten.

Von

Dr. S. Goldflam,
Warschau.

Im Jahre 1891 habe ich eine Beobachtung von Bulbärlähmung mit Ergriffensein der Extremitäten veröffentlicht, die dadurch ausgezeichnet war, dass Genesung eintrat.[1]) In der letzten Zeit hatte ich 3 derartige Fälle zu beobachten Gelegenheit; sie scheinen darzuthun, dass die schlimme Prognose des bulbärparalytischen Symptomencomplexes eine Einschränkung erheischt, und dass es sich wahrscheinlich um eine eigenartige Erkrankung handelt.

Fall 1. Johann O..., 25 Jahre alt, Hausdiener, kam am 22. December 1891 in meine Poliklinik zur Behandlung. Seine Krankheit begann vor 7 Wochen mit Taubheitsgefühl im Nacken, Beschränkung der Kopfbewegungen, Kopfschmerzen, Schwindel beim Bücken. Schon nach einer Woche traten Sprach- und Schluckstörungen hinzu, dann Schwäche in den Armen, nach ein paar Tagen auch in den Beinen. In den letzteren, in den Schultern und der Kreuzgegend empfand er reissende Schmerzen. Nach Verlauf von 2 Wochen steigerte sich die Gliederschwäche derart, dass der Kranke das Bett aufsuchen musste, in welchem er sich nur mühsam umzudrehen vermochte, den Kopf gar nicht bewegen konnte und gefüttert werden musste. In diesem hülflosen Zustande lag er 2 Wochen zu Hause, ebensoviel Zeit in einem Krankenhause. Zu dieser Zeit, also ungefähr 6 Wochen nach Beginn der Krankheit, fing eine Besserung sich einzustellen, der Pat. konnte kurz darauf das Krankenhaus verlassen. Stuhlverstopfung begleitete den ganzen bisherigen Verlauf der Krankheit, in deren Beginne Fieber vorhanden gewesen sein soll; doch ist diese letzte Angabe des Kranken unsicher.

Er war immer gesund, hat Syphilis nicht überstanden, keine Excesse in Baccho et Venere geübt; Intoxication mit Blei, anderen Metallen und Substanzen, Diphtherie konnten entschieden ausgeschlossen werden.

Es ist ein Mann von mässigem Wuchse, normalem Körperbau und gut entwickelter Musculatur, Hautfarbe blass, Puls 90, Respiration 18, innere

1) Neurolog. Centralbl. 1891. Nr. 6 u. 7.

After thoroughly describing his three cases and reviewing the past medical literature, including Erb's cases, Goldflam concluded:

"The compiled material presented here appears sufficient to prove that cases with bulbar symptom complex exist which do not fit the known categories. They form a closely related group which differs from other bulbar affections in general physical appearance of the disease, in method of development and type of symptoms, in distinct prognosis and negative anatomical findings. Therefore, it deserves a unique position as a distinct disease entity."

Since Goldflam encountered all three of his cases in a brief span of time, he speculated that they were caused by the effect of an infectious toxin upon the brain.

His summary of the characteristic findings of what became known as the "Erb-Goldflam Symptom-Complex" outlines the main features of this condition:

Henry Viets, founder of the first Myasthenia Gravis Clinic in the United States at Boston's Massachusetts General Hospital in 1935, claimed that Goldflam's paper was "the most important ever written in the history of the disease."[3]

"The question whether a diagnosis of this primary and in some cases curable malady is possible must be answered affirmatively when bulbar symptoms in a young individual occur in rather rapid succession and trunk and extremities are also involved in the weakness; when the bulbar paralysis differs in many respects from that of Duchenne; when the masseter muscles are affected early and severely in addition to the lower and upper face regions; when ptosis or paresis of the extraocular muscles is present, but atrophy, fibrillary spasms or changes in electrical excitability are absent; when respiratory complaints and attacks of dyspnea play an important role in the picture of the disease and the weakness exhibits the above-mentioned characteristics; when it deals with rapid and easily occurring fatigue of the muscles; when the symptoms fluctuate not only from day to day but also during the course of a day; when considerable remissions and exacerbations occur and the tendon reflexes are normal; then we deal with the species of disease discussed here."

(English translations by Karin I. Molnar, with permission)

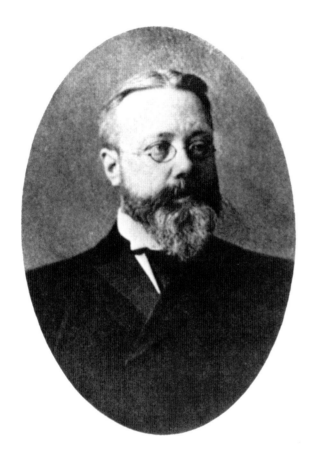

Friedrich Jolly, 1895

A little over a year after Goldflam's paper appeared, the term "myasthenia gravis pseudoparalytica" was introduced in December 1894 at a lecture to the Berlin Medical Society by Friedrich Jolly, recently appointed instead of Oppenheim to be Carl Friederich Otto Westphal's successor as director of the clinic at the Charité in Berlin.

At the lecture Jolly demonstrated the rapid but reversible fatigue of the limbs of a 14-year-old boy, and also showed smoked drum tracings of the responses of the boy's leg muscles to continuous faradic tetanization, "whether it be the nerves or directly" (?), compared to those of a person without the condition.

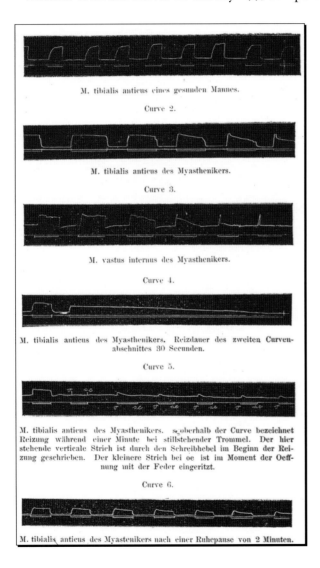

M. tibialis anticus eines gesunden Mannes.

Curve 2.

M. tibialis anticus des Myasthenikers.

Curve 3.

M. vastus internus des Myasthenikers.

Curve 4.

M. tibialis anticus des Myasthenikers. Reizdauer des zweiten Curven-abschnittes 30 Secunden.

Curve 5.

M. tibialis anticus des Myasthenikers. s oberhalb der Curve bezeichnet Reizung während einer Minute bei stillstehender Trommel. Der hier stehende verticale Strich ist durch den Schreibhebel im Beginn der Reizung geschrieben. Der kleinere Strich bei oe ist im Moment der Oeffnung mit der Feder eingeritzt.

Curve 6.

M. tibialis anticus des Myastenikers nach einer Ruhepause von 2 Minuten.

The **first curve** is taken from the *m. tibialis anticus* of the healthy man. It shows that during the entire period of stimulation, the maximum, achieved earlier, continues. With termination of the stimulus, the curve falls off abruptly. With a new stimulus, it returns to the same height up until the end of the stimulus, describing a very nearly horizontal line. (The small peaks and troughs throughout the curve come from fibrillary undulations, such as those which one often sees during the application of tetanizing current during the strong contraction of muscles.) In healthy individuals we can administer such stimuli, one after the other, without any change.

The latter appear quite different in the sick muscles of our patient, as is visible in curves 2 and 3, wherein the second is also of the *tibialis anticus*, while the third is of the *vastus internus*.

Curve 2 shows, at the first stimulus, the almost horizontal course of the curve, at the second, a noticeable downstroke, at the third a very significant downstroke, and after the fourth stimulus, after a rather short up-swing, there is a sudden downstroke, then a slow downstroke, and upon the fifth stimulus, the beginning upstroke falls even more rapidly and precipitously at the second portion of the curve.

Curve 3 shows even more clearly a precipitous dropoff at the third stimulus; by the fourth, the beginning tick with subsequent drop-off falls almost to the zero line; by the fifth, a more noticeably reduced beginning tick; after the dropoff, only a minimal contraction is evident.

In curves 4, 5, and 6, curves also from the *tibialis anticus* have been reproduced. Curve 4 shows the normal curve of the tetanus during the course of a brief stimulus, followed by, upon continuation for about a half minute, a similar gradual decrease, until it disappears completely. After a pause of 2 minutes, curve 5 was obtained, which demonstrates, once again, the continuing tetanus during stimulation, then, after about 2 seconds, at the letter S, stimulation occurred. At the same time, the drum was stopped and only set in motion again at the conclusion of the stimulus. Then, at ö, the current was interrupted. During the stimulus, the device's arm had already sunk to the zero line. The subsequent stimuli had only an initial twitch, no more tetanus as a result. After the muscle had been granted a respite of about 2 minutes, in order to recover, curve 6 was drawn, which demonstrates the gradual transition into flat contraction with initial twitches, without, during the time the drum was turning, the tetanus having disappeared entirely.

Curve 4. *M. tibialis anticus* of a person with myasthenia. Stimulus duration of the second portion of the curve is about 30 seconds.

Curve 5. *M. tibialis anticus* of a person with myasthenia. The stimulus described about the curve was from one minute with the drum standing still. The vertical stroke was produced by the writing arm at the beginning of the stimulus. The smaller stroke by ö is inscribed at the outset by the recording arm.

Curve 6. *M. tibialis anticus* of a person with myasthenia after a pause of 2 minutes.

(English translation by Ron Hay)

Jolly called the decline of the stimulated muscle response "the myasthenic reaction." "Myasthenia" was a term for muscular debility. Jolly thought that the cause of the fatigue resided in the muscle but that more of the central nervous system than just the "bulb" might also be involved. He therefore objected to terms which emphasized the bulbar aspects, and suggested instead the term "myasthenia gravis pseudoparalytica," adding the word "generalisata" where appropriate. Jolly published his lecture and demonstration in 1895 with the title "Ueber Myasthenia gravis pseudoparalytica."[4]

Summary

By the turn of the century some sixty cases of this distinct syndrome had been reported from a variety of European countries and even from America and Moscow, although there was no agreement about the most appropriate name for the condition.

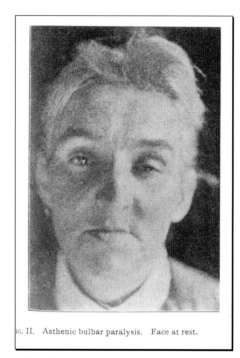

IG. II. Asthenic bulbar paralysis.   Face at rest.

This photograph of a person with myasthenia gravis appeared in an 1899 article by **Wharton Sinkler** of Philadelphia, Pennsylvania[5] on "Asthenic bulbar paralysis," a term introduced by von Strumpell in 1896.

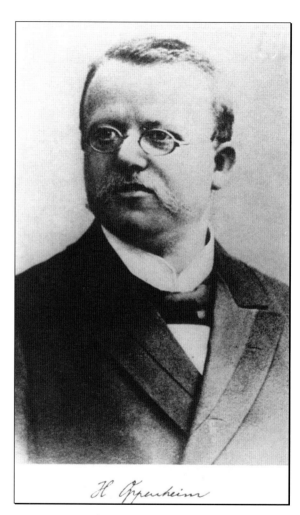

Herman Oppenheim, whose private clinic in Berlin became an international center of clinical neurology, summarized 58 of these cases in his important 1901 monograph, *Die Myasthenische Paralyse (Bulbarparalyse ohne anatomischen Befund)* in 1901.[6]

THE PRINCIPLES AND
PRACTICE OF MEDICINE

DESIGNED FOR THE USE OF PRACTITIONERS
AND STUDENTS OF MEDICINE

BY

WILLIAM OSLER, M. D.

Fellow of the Royal Society; Fellow of the Royal College of Physicians,
London; Professor of Medicine in the Johns Hopkins University and
Physician-in-chief to the Johns Hopkins Hospital, Baltimore;
formerly Professor of the Institutes of Medicine, McGill
University, Montreal; and Professor of Clinical Medicine
in the University of Pennsylvania, Philadelphia

THIRD EDITION

NEW YORK
D. APPLETON AND COMPANY
1899

---

6. ASTHENIC (BULBAR) PARALYSIS

(*Myasthenia gravis pseudo-paralytica*; *Erb-Goldflam's Symptom-complex*).

During the last few years much attention has been given to this remarkable affection, of which a number of cases have been reported. The chief characteristics are the rapidity with which the muscles become exhausted, the great variability of the symptoms from day to day, the occurrence of remissions and relapses, the sudden attacks of paralysis of respiration and deglutition, and the absence of muscular atrophy, the reaction of degeneration and sensory symptoms. The onset is usually acute or subacute, chiefly in young persons. The external eye muscles, the muscles of mastication, the facial muscles, the muscles of deglutition, and certain spinal muscles may be quickly involved. Any repeated efforts with the affected muscles causes them to become completely exhausted and paralyzed for the time being. They recover their power after a rest. In certain cases there is a true paresis, which persists. After repeated stimulation by electricity the muscles may become exhausted and cease to respond (myasthenic reaction, Golly). The affection may prove fatal, and as no well-defined anatomical lesions have been discovered, a dynamic change in the lower motor neurones has been assumed to explain the condition.

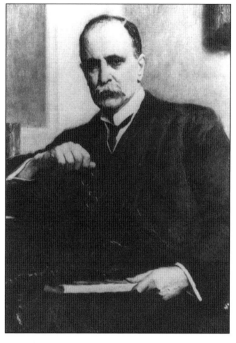

William Osler, professor of medicine at the Johns Hopkins University and physician-in-chief to the Johns Hopkins Hospital in Baltimore, Maryland, chose "Asthenic (Bulbar) Paralysis" as the favored term for the third edition in 1899 of his textbook, The *Principles and Practice of Medicine,* but by the fourth edition in 1901 he preferred "Myasthenia Gravis."

THE PRINCIPLES AND
PRACTICE OF MEDICINE

DESIGNED FOR THE USE OF PRACTITIONERS
AND STUDENTS OF MEDICINE

BY

WILLIAM OSLER, M. D.

Fellow of the Royal Society; Fellow of the Royal College of Physicians,
London; Professor of Medicine in the Johns Hopkins University and
Physician-in-chief to the Johns Hopkins Hospital, Baltimore;
formerly Professor of the Institutes of Medicine, McGill
University, Montreal; and Professor of Clinical Medicine
in the University of Pennsylvania, Philadelphia

FOURTH EDITION

NEW YORK
D. APPLETON AND COMPANY
1901

---

6. MYASTHENIA GRAVIS

(*Asthenic Bulbar Paralysis*; *Erb-Goldflam's Symptom-complex*).

Some sixty cases are on record and have been analyzed by Harry Campbell and Edwin Bramwell (Brain, 1901). The etiology is unknown. Young persons are chiefly affected. The muscles innervated by the bulb are first affected—those of the eyes, the face, of mastication, and of the neck. All the voluntary muscles may become involved. After rest the power is recovered. In severe cases paralysis may persist. The myasthenic reaction of Jolly is the rapid exhaustion of the muscles, by faradism, not by galvanism. There are marked remissions and fluctuations in the severity of the symptoms. The affected muscles in a few cases have atrophied. Of 17 autopsies, in only 6 was anything abnormal found (C. and B.), and the significance of the changes is doubtful.

The diagnosis is easy—from the ptosis, the facial expression, the nasal speech, the rapid fatigue of the muscles, the myasthenic reaction, the absence of atrophy, tremors, etc., and the remarkable variations in the intensity of the symptoms. Of the 60 cases, 23 ended fatally. The patient may live many years; recovery may take place. Rest, strychnia in full doses, massage, alternate courses of iodide of potassium and mercury may be tried.

In Retrospect

Once the clinical syndrome of myasthenia gravis had been thoroughly described and accepted, isolated earlier examples of what might have been myasthenia were proposed as being the first described case. Oosterhuis discovered that the French clinician **M. Hérard** had described a convincing case in 1868 which was considered at the time to be an uncommon variant of "la paralysie glosso-labiolaryngée,"[7] while Goldflam had noted the brief account by **Samuel Wilks**, English physician to Guy's Hospital in London, published in 1877.

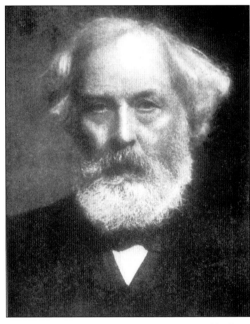

Samuel Wilks described several cases of bulbar paralysis in 1877, in one of which no disease was found at autopsy.[8]

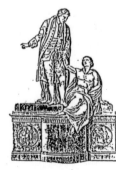

GUY'S HOSPITAL REPORTS.

EDITED BY
H. G. HOWSE, M.S.,
AND
FREDERICK TAYLOR, M.D.

Third Series.
VOL. XXII.

LONDON:
J. & A. CHURCHILL, NEW BURLINGTON STREET.

MDCCCLXXVII.

ON
CEREBRITIS, HYSTERIA, AND BULBAR PARALYSIS,
AS ILLUSTRATIVE OF
ARREST OF FUNCTION OF THE CEREBRO-SPINAL CENTRES.

BY SAMUEL WILKS, M.D.

CASE. *Bulbar paralysis; fatal; no disease found.*—A stout girl, looking well, came to the hospital on account of general weakness; she could scarcely walk or move about, she spoke slowly and had slight strabismus. The house-physician was inclined to regard the case as one of hysteria; as he possessed a special knowledge of eye affections, he saw nothing in the strabismus incompatible with this view. She remained in this state about a month, being neither better nor worse; she was able to walk about, but every movement of her limbs and speech was performed so slowly and deliberately that the case seemed rather one of lethargy from want of will than an actual paralysis. At the end of this period all the symptoms became aggravated, and in about three days they had assumed all the well-marked characters of bulbar paralysis. She spoke most indistinctly, swallowed with great difficulty, and was quite unable to cough. The limbs were, however not paralysed, as she was able to get out of her bed. It was shortly afterwards seen that her respiration was becoming affected, the difficulty of which rapidly increased, and in a few hours she died. The medulla oblongata was very carefully examined, and no disease was found. It appeared quite healthy to the naked eye, and the microscope discovered no manifest change in the tissue.

In 1903 Guthrie[9] resurrected, as the first case of myasthenia, that described in 1672 by **Thomas Willis**, an eminent London physician who had been Professor of Natural History at Oxford University. The 1672 Latin treatise, *De Anima Brutorum*,[10] was translated into English by Pordage in 1683 as "The London Practice of Physick, or the Whole Practical Part of Physick Contained in the Works of Dr. Willis."[11]

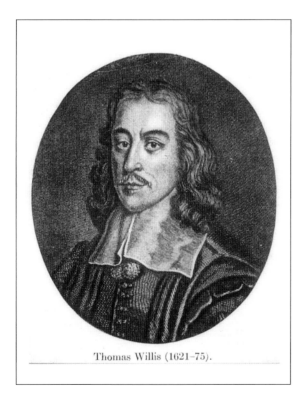

Thomas Willis (1621–75).

ther they can go or not; Nevertheless, those labouring with a want of Spirits, who will exercife local motions, as well as they can, in the morning are able to walk firmly, to fling about their Arms hither and thither, or to take up any heavy thing; before noon the ftock of the Spirits being fpent, which had flowed into the Mufcles, they are fcarce able to move Hand or Foot. At this time I have under my charge a prudent and an honeft Woman, who for many years hath been obnoxious to this fort of fpurious *Palfie*, not only in her Members, but alfo in her tongue; fhe fo fome time can fpeak freely and readily enough, but after fhe has fpoke long, or haftily, or eagerly, fhe is not able to fpeak a word, but becomes as mute as a Fifh, nor can fhe recover the ufe of her voice under an hour or two.

Excerpt from Pordage's 1683 English translation describing Willis's case of "The Spurious Palsy."

T hen in 1988 Marstellar[12] proposed that perhaps the Indian chief **Opechankanough**, 28 years before Willis's description, might have had myasthenia to explain why a formerly vigorous man developed ptosis and fluctuating weakness and had to be carried into battle by his warriors in 1644. These interesting speculations, however, should not detract from the clinical descriptions of myasthenia gravis initiated by Erb and Goldflam in the German medical literature.

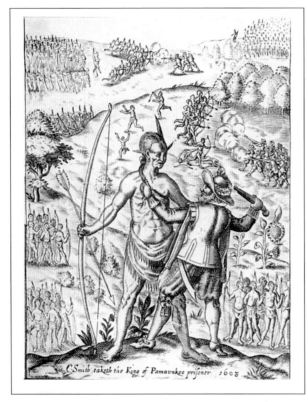

Captain John Smith threatening the impressive and apparently vigorous Indian Chief Opechankanough in 1608 (from Bridenbaugh, C., *Early Americans*, New York, Oxford University Press, 1981).

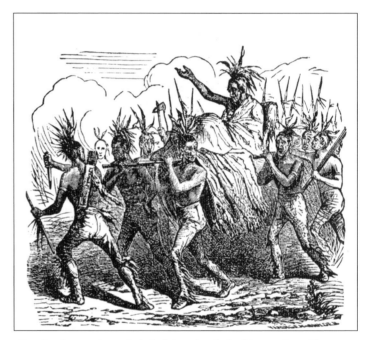

Opechankanough carried aloft into battle by his warriors. Note his weakened appearance and his ptosis.[12]

References for Chapter 1: Clinical Recognition (1879-1901)

1. Erb W: Sur Casuistik der bulbären Lähmungen. *Archiv für Psychiatrie und Nervenkrankheiten* 9:336-350, 1879.

2. Goldflam S: Ueber einen scheinbar heilbaren bulbärparalytischen Symptomencomplex mit Betheiligung der Extremitäten. *Deutsche Zeitschrift für Nervenheilkunde* 4:312-352, 1893.

3. Viets HR: A historical review of myasthenia gravis from 1672 to 1900. *J American Medical Association* 153:1273-1280, 1953.

4. Jolly FI: Ueber Myasthenia gravis pseudoparalytica. *Berliner Klinische Wochenschrift* 32:1-7, 1895.

5. Sinkler W: Asthenic bulbar paralysis. *J Nervous & Mental Disease* 26:536-544, 1899.

6. Oppenheim H: *Die Myasthenische Paralyse (Bulbarparalyse ohne anatomischen Befund)*, Berlin, Germany: JHH Karger, 1901.

7. cited in Oosterhuis HJGH: *Myasthenia Gravis*. Edinburgh, Scotland: Churchill Livingstone, 1984.

8. Wilks S: On cerebritis, hysteria, and bulbar paralysis. *Guy's Hospital Reports* 22:7-55, 1877.

9. Guthrie LG: "Myasthenia Gravis" in the seventeenth century. *Lancet* 1:330-331, 1903.

10. Willis T: *De anima brutorum quae hominis vitalis ac sensitiva est, exercitations duae*. Oxford, England: Londini, Typis EF, impensis Ric Davis, 1672.

11. Willis T: *Two discourses concerning the soul of brutes, which is that of the vital and sensitive of man*. In: Pordage S, trans: *The London Practice of Physick, or the Whole Practical Part of Physick Contained in the Works of Dr. Willis*. London, England: printed for Thomas Bassett and William Crooke, pp. 431-432, 1685.

12. Marstellar HB: The first American case of myasthenia gravis. *Archives of Neurology* 45:185-187, 1988.

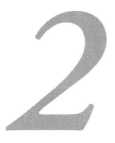

The Search for Morbid Anatomy (1901-1966)

Introduction

The new scientific approach to neurological disease, championed by Charcot in France, emphasized not only precision of clinical observation (which was the subject of the former chapter) but also exactitude of anatomical analysis. At the turn of the century the anatomy of organs or tissues in a state of disease was termed "morbid anatomy." Early investigators looked at the central nervous system for explanations for the clinical aspects of myasthenia gravis because of its similarities with progressive bulbar paralysis mentioned above, but no appropriate lesions could be found in either the brain or brainstem in myasthenia gravis. However, complete examination revealed occasional abnormalities in the thymus gland, a structure of then-unknown function which is located underneath the breastbone and above the heart in a region known as the anterior mediastinum.

Early Studies Concerning The Thymus in Myasthenia Gravis

In 1899 Oppenheim reported as an incidental finding the presence of a tumor "the size of a mandarin orange" growing from the thymic remnant of a patient who died with myasthenia gravis.

When one of the leading pathologists of his time, **Carl Weigert**, described in 1901 the autopsy findings[1] of a case of "Erb's Disease (Myasthenia gravis)" reported by Leopold Laquer[2] from Frankfurt, he noted that the central nervous system was normal but an invasive tumor of thymic origin was present in the anterior mediastinum. The tumor was made up of white blood cells called lymphoid cells, conspicuous collections of which Weigert also found present in the deltoid and diaphragm muscles as well as in heart muscle. He concluded that these were metastases from the malignant thymic tumor, which he thus interpreted as a lymphosarcoma.

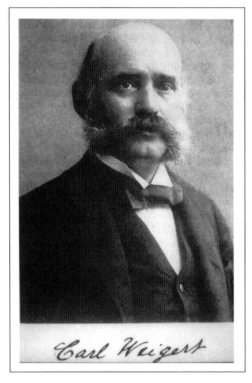

Carl Weigert

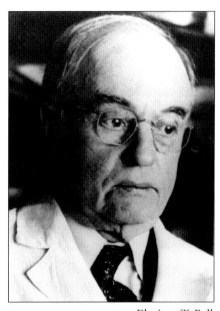
Elexious T. Bell

In a review by **Elexious T. Bell**, professor of pathology at the University of Minnesota, of 56 autopsies performed on patients with myasthenia gravis between 1901 and 1917, the thymus was described as "enlarged" in 17 and contained a tumor in ten others.[3] Bell agreed with James Ewing's suggestion of the year before (1916) that the most suitable term to describe these tumors was "thymoma." But Bell also noted that in 17 similar autopsies reported on patients with myasthenia gravis before 1900 the thymus was not mentioned. Therefore he concluded that *"thymic lesions cannot be regarded as the cause of myasthenia, since they are present in only about half the cases."*

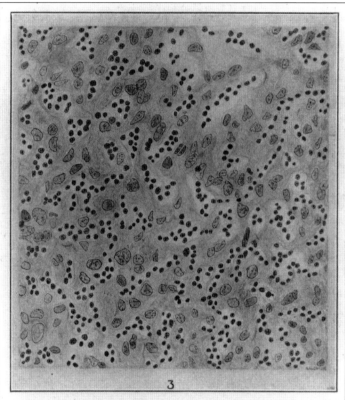

FIG. 3. A typical area of the tumor showing the epithelial reticulum and numerous lymphocytes in the spaces. This corresponds to the structure of the fetal thymus at the stage of the lymphoid transformation. Drawing. × 600.

A drawing of the microscopic appearance of a thymoma, from Bell's 1917 paper.

However, by the time **Edgar Hughes Norris**, also then a professor of pathology from the University of Minnesota, published his review[4] of the pathology of myasthenia gravis in 1936, almost twenty years after Bell but still before successful surgical removal of the thymus, he could state that "pathologic changes may be found in the thymus in cases of myasthenia gravis in direct ratio to the care with which they are sought." These consisted of "greater or less degrees of epithelial hyperplasia" (cellularity) on microscopic examination, thymomas being considered examples of "a marked degree of hyperplasia."

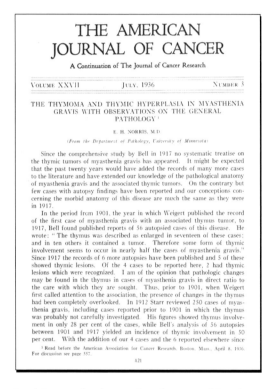

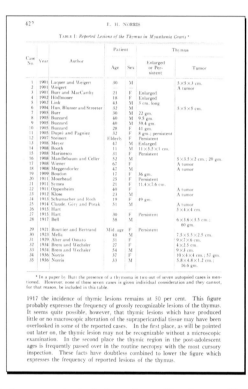

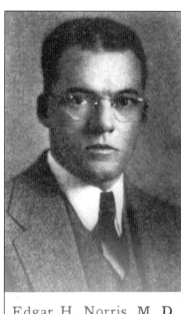

Edgar H. Norris, M. D.

Despite his emphasis on the thymus, Norris nevertheless concluded that the collections of lymphoid cells in muscles, first noted by Weigert in 1901 and found in two-thirds of autopsied cases of myasthenia gravis by 1936, were more characteristic of myasthenia gravis than the changes found in the thymus.

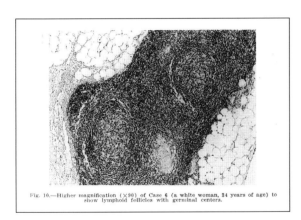

Fig. 10.—Higher magnification (×90) of Case 6 (a white woman, 34 years of age) to show lymphoid follicles with germinal centers.

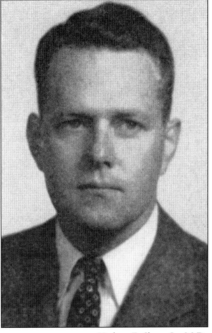

Herbert E. Sloan, Jr., M.D.

The distinguishing pathological feature of the non-tumorous thymus apparently escaped detection until 1943 when **Herbert Sloan**, a Fellow in Surgery at Johns Hopkins University, first described the fact that the medulla (or central part) of the thymus in patients with MG contained numerous "lymphoid follicles with germinal centers." A germinal center is the central portion of a nodule of lymphocytes, the characteristic feature of lymph nodes. Germinal centers are usually not present in the normal thymus. It turns out that myasthenia is not unique in having germinal centers in the thymus, but they are much more frequent in myasthenia than in other conditions.

Recent Advances in Surgery

CONDUCTED BY ALFRED BLALOCK, M.D.

THE THYMUS IN MYASTHENIA GRAVIS

WITH OBSERVATIONS ON THE NORMAL ANATOMY AND HISTOLOGY OF THE THYMUS

HERBERT E. SLOAN, JR., M.D.,* BALTIMORE, MD.

(From the Departments of Surgery and Pathology of the Johns Hopkins University)

BLALOCK, Harvey, Ford, and Lilienthal[1] have reported the effects of removing the thymus from six patients with myasthenia gravis; more recently Blalock has removed the thymus from four additional patients. The diagnosis in each case was confirmed by the response to prostigmine salts and the intra-arterial injection of prostigmine methylsulfate. Stimulated by the marked improvement in some of these cases following operation, an investigation of the pathology of the thymus in myasthenia gravis was begun. None of the ten operative specimens examined contained a tumor. In order to establish a basis for comparison 350 thymus glands were examined between August 5, 1941, and March 23, 1942. These included approximately 200 specimens removed during routine autopsies at the Johns Hopkins Hospital and 150 specimens removed from patients who died suddenly and were autopsied at the city morgue.[†]

EMBRYOLOGY AND HISTOLOGY

It is usually stated that during the sixth week of embryonic life the thymus arises as ventral, cylindrical outgrowths of the third pair of pharyngeal pouches. These hollow epithelial cylinders, arising from the entoderm, soon elongate, become solid, and enlarge at their free ends. Simultaneously, parathyroid III arises from the dorsal diverticulum of the third pharyngeal pouch. During this process the mesial portions of the pharyngeal pouches, lying between these structures and the pharynx, atrophy and disappear. Thus, the two lobes of the thymus, accompanied by the detached cervical sinus, and the two parathyroids become independent structures. The caudal end of the thymus enlarges. With the great vessels and the heart, the thymus and parathyroid III move caudally towards the thorax. Parathyroid III normally ceases its descent near the lower pole of the thyroid, the thymus separating from it as it progresses into the thorax. The two lobes extend over

*William Stewart Halsted Fellow in Surgery.
†Dr. W. G. VandeGrift, assistant medical examiner, made it possible for these specimens to be obtained.

154

Pathology of Muscle in Myasthenia Gravis – "Lymphorrhages"

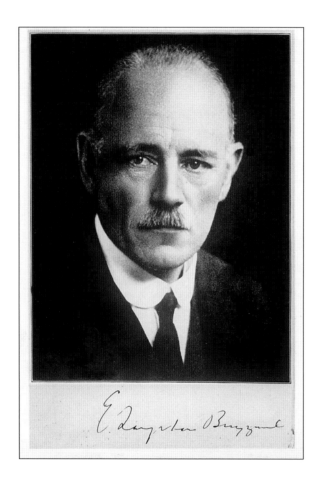

In 1905, four years after Weigert's report, **E. Farquhar Buzzard**, a prominent London neurologist, described lymphoid deposits which he termed "lymphorrhages" in muscles, adrenal glands, heart, liver and thyroid gland, but not in the brain or spinal cord, of five autopsy cases of myasthenia gravis, not all of which had thymic abnormalities.[5]

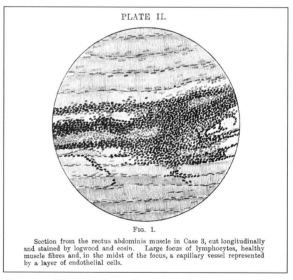

PLATE II.

FIG. 1.

Section from the rectus abdominis muscle in Case 3, cut longitudinally and stained by logwood and eosin. Large focus of lymphocytes, healthy muscle fibres and, in the midst of the focus, a capillary vessel represented by a layer of endothelial cells.

Drawing of lymphorrhages from Buzzard's 1905 paper.

Buzzard said, *"My cases show that abnormalities of the thymus are not constant features in this disease, and therefore that the lymphocytic deposits which occur independently of them are probably not in any way a secondary condition. On the other hand my experience affords reasonable grounds for believing that lymphorrhages are constantly present in the muscles or other organs in cases of myasthenia. That they existed in all five of my cases was only established by a diligent search through some thousands of sections, and for that reason it would be unwise to assume that they were absent from the cases of other observers who had not been led to conduct a similar careful investigation with the same object."*

Buzzard concluded that the cells in lymphorrhages came from blood vessels and that the symptoms of the disease were best explained by the presence of some "toxic, possibly autotoxic, agent which has a special influence on the protoplasmic constituent of voluntary muscle."

THE CLINICAL HISTORY AND *POST-MORTEM* EXAMINATION OF FIVE CASES OF MYASTHENIA GRAVIS.

BY E. FARQUHAR BUZZARD, M.D., M.R.C.P.,

Assistant Physician to the National Hospital for the Paralysed and Epileptic, to the Royal Free Hospital, and to the Belgrave Hospital for Children.

With Five Figures.

IN a paper which was read before the Pathological Society of London I have already given a short summary of the histological findings in the five cases of myasthenia gravis which form the subject of this communication, but it appears to me desirable that a full account of these cases should be placed on record, inasmuch as they present features which are not only of pathological but of clinical interest.

The object of the present paper may therefore be regarded as two-fold. In the first place it will draw attention to some striking clinical phenomena occasionally occurring in this disease, and in the second place it will serve to propagate the view, which my experience has caused me to hold, that there are constant morbid changes associated with myasthenia gravis.

My best thanks are due to Dr. T. Buzzard, Dr. Ormerod, Dr. Head, and Dr. Wall, for their kind permission to make use of the clinical notes on the cases under their care.

Case 1.—A. J., aged 41, was admitted into the National Hospital under the care of Dr. T. Buzzard on November 3, 1903. His family history was too vague to be of importance.

His previous health had been good ; but at 16 he contracted gonorrhœa, followed by no evidence of a sore or of secondary syphilitic symptoms. In 1892 he injured left eye and suffered from monocular diplopia for eight years. Moderate drinker of beer ; no spirits. Occupation for twenty-one years had been that of a stone-grainer. Married nineteen years ; fourteen children, of whom six died in infancy and one was stillborn.

The microscopic appearance of muscles from patients with myasthenia gravis was still of interest in 1953 when **Dorothy Russell** in London noted that lymphorrhages were one of three types of similar muscle abnormalities found in eight cases of myasthenia gravis.[6] Russell concluded that these changes might be important regarding the weakness characteristic of myasthenia, but that they were not peculiar to myasthenia gravis and therefore not diagnostic of the condition. Even today the significance of lymphorrhages is still uncertain.

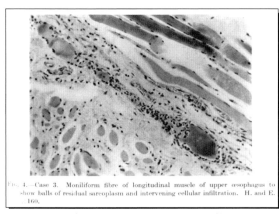

Type I change from Russell's 1953 paper with fiber necrosis.

The Journal of

Pathology and Bacteriology

Vol. LXV, No. 2

HISTOLOGICAL CHANGES IN THE STRIPED
MUSCLES IN MYASTHENIA GRAVIS

Dorothy S. Russell

*From the Bernhard Baron Institute of Pathology,
The London Hospital*

Summary

Three types of histological change are described in the striped muscle fibres in a series of eight cases of myasthenia gravis.

Type I is an acute change in which fibres undergo necrosis, with resulting inflammatory cellular reaction, and disappear.

Type II is a progressive atrophy of individual fibres associated, in the later stages, with the formation of lymphorrhages.

Type III is a simple atrophy of different character from that of type II; it affects single fibres or groups of fibres.

The incidence and distribution of these types are analysed in the different muscles studied in the eight cases. The results appear similar whether there is a thymic tumour (four cases) or not.

It is concluded that the changes are important in relation to the clinical evidence of muscular dysfunction. They are not, however, peculiar to myasthenia gravis and are not, therefore, diagnostic of this condition.

Type III change was not illustrated.

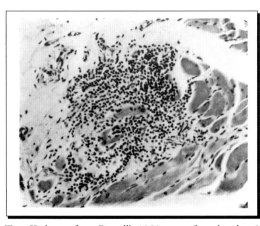

Type II change from Russell's 1953 paper (lymphorrhage).

The Presence of Myoid Cells in the Thymus – Important in Myasthenia?

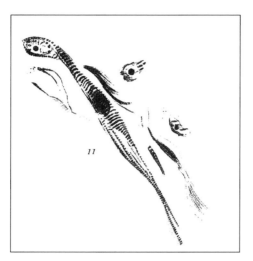

Cells in the thymus with striations similar to those found in striated muscles (the kind of muscles affected in myasthenia gravis) were first noted in the frog thymus by **Sigmund Mayer** of Prague in 1888 and termed "myoidzellen" (myoid cells) by **J. A. Hammar** from Uppsala, Sweden, in 1910. Also in 1910, elongated myoid cells with striations (illustrated on left) were described for the first time in the thymus of a 5 1/2-month *human* fetus, by **Alvin Pappenheimer** of Bellevue Hospital in New York City.[7]

However, these cells were believed to disappear from the thymus during maturation. Their presence was generally overlooked until the 1960's when proteins in the sera from some myasthenic patients, especially those with thymomas, were found to attach to cells in the thymus as well as to striated muscle cells (See Chapter 4, page 51). The interest in thymic myoid cells was revived especially when in 1966 they were found in the thymuses of adult patients with myasthenia gravis by **Robert Van de Velde** and **Nathan Friedman** of Cedars-Sinai Medical Center, Los Angeles.[8] However, more recently myoid cells have also been found in the thymuses of humans without myasthenia, so their significance, like that of lymphorrhages, is presently unclear.

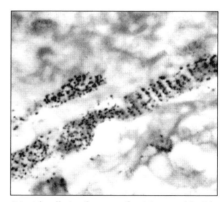

Myoid cells in thymus of a 16-year-old girl with very severe form of myasthenia gravis. (Modified Bodian's Protargol stain. X 800.)

The Junction Between the Nerve Ending and the Muscle Fiber

Thymic tumors, lymphorrhages and thymic myoid cells, although tantalizing, have so far failed to explain the pathophysiology of myasthenia gravis. Evidence in subsequent chapters will point to the place where the motor nerve meets the muscle fiber as the most likely location of the immediate pathology in myasthenia gravis, but in the early days of the search for "morbid anatomy," this myoneural junction (also called the neuromuscular junction) was a very poorly understood structure.

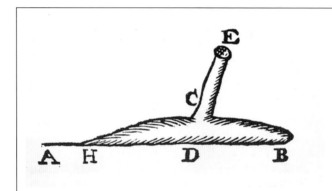

Herman Boerhaave of Leyden, the 18th century founder of Dutch medicine, believed that the nerve (EC in the 1743 illustration above) flowed directly into the substance of the muscle HB. (Boerhaave, Institutiones medicae, page 91, Leyden, 1734)[9]

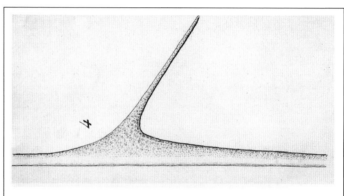

Even one hundred years later, in 1840, the magnifying power of contemporary light microscopes was such that the two structures were still pictured as fused,[10] as in the neuromuscular junction of a microscopic animal called a tardigrade (above).

The fine structure of the myoneural junction was apparently beyond the capabilities of the finest light microscopists. One of these, **Willy Kühne,** Director of the Institute of Physiology at Heidelberg, published this remarkable drawing in 1863 of the side view of a nerve ending on a guinea pig muscle.[11] Below it is a 1976 photo taken through a Nomarski interference contrast microscope.[12] The similarities between Kühne's drawing and the modern photomicrograph are striking, but the nature of the junction is still indistinct.

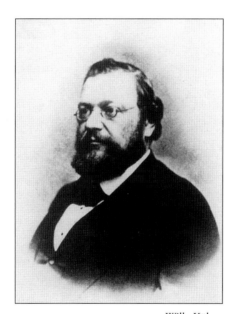

Willy Kühne

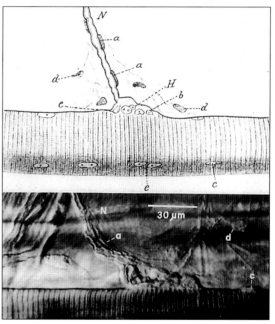

Side view of single living guinea pig endplates. Top: M. gastrocnemius (Kühne, 1863). Bottom: M. sternocleidomastoideus pars clavicularis. Nomarski interference contrast (40 x water immersion lens). *N* nerve, *a* Schwann cell nuclei, *H* nuclei in and at endplate, *c* muscle nuclei, *d* collagen nuclei[12] (reprinted with permission from Springer-Verlag).

Photomicrographs of motor nerve endings, and the muscle end plates underlying them, obtained by biopsy from living patients with myasthenia gravis and stained with intravital methylene blue, were thought by some observers in 1958 to be more elongated with less side-branching than normal endplates. These were termed "dysplastic" by **C. Coërs** and **J.E. Desmedt** of Brussels, Belgium, who perfected this technique.[13]

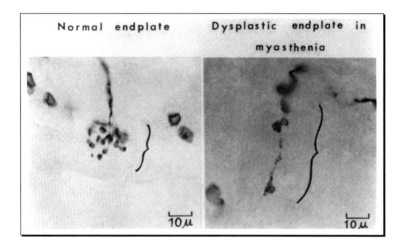

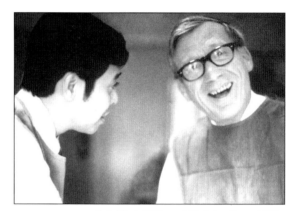

Luis Chui, M.D., and Christian Coërs, M.D.,
Los Angeles County Medical Center, 1972

Stronger magnification was needed to elucidate what might be wrong at the neuromuscular junction in MG, such as might be provided by the electron microscope. Although the principles of the electron microscope and a few prototypes were available in the 1930's, the electron microscope did not become commercially available until after World War II. Even then, however, the early evidence from the electron microscope of the location of the neuromuscular pathology in myasthenia gravis would continue to be controversial, as we shall see.

BUT FIRST WE NEED TO FOLLOW a *functional* trail to the neuromuscular junction provided by the use of substances that had been obtained from various plants.

References for Chapter 2: The Search for Morbid Anatomy (1901-1966)

1. Weigert C: Pathologisch-anatomischer Beiträg zur Erb'schen Krankheit (Myasthenia gravis). *Neurologisches Zentralblatt* 20:597-601, 1901.

2. Laquer L: Ueber die Erb'sche Krankeit (Myasthenia gravis). *Neurologisches Zentralblatt* 20:594-596, 1901.

3. Bell ET: Tumors of the thymus in myasthenia gravis. *J Nervous & Mental Diseases* 45:130-143, 1917.

4. Norris EH: The thymoma and thymic hyperplasia in myasthenia gravis with observations on the general pathology. *American J Cancer* 27:421-433, 1936.

5. Buzzard EF: The clinical history and post-mortem examination of five cases of myasthenia gravis. *Brain* 28:438-483, 1905.

6. Russell DS: Histological changes in the striped muscles in myasthenia gravis. *J Pathology and Bacteriology* 65:279-289, 1953.

7. Pappenheimer AM: A contribution to the normal and pathological histology of the thymus gland. *J of Medical Research* 22:1-73, 1910.

8. Van de Velde RL, Friedman NB: Thymic myoid cells and myasthenia gravis. *American J Pathology* 59:347-367, 1970.

9. cited in Brazier MAB: *A History of Neurophysiology in the 17th and 18th Centuries, From Concept to Experiment* p. 114. Raven Press, New York, 1984.

10. Doyère M: Mémoire sur les Tardigrades. *Annales des Sciences Naturelles* 14:269-351, 1840.

11. Kühne W: Uber die peripherischen Endogane der motorischen Nerven, Mit 5 Tafeln. Leipzig, W. Engelmann, 1863.

12. Dreyer F, Müller K-D, Peper K, Sterz R: The M. omohyoideus of the mouse as a convenient mammalian muscle preparation. *Pflugers Archiv* 367:115-122, 1976.

13. Coërs C, Desmedt J: Abnormal end-plates in myasthenic muscle. *Lancet* 2:1124, 1958.

3 From Plants to Materia Medica (1927-1935)

Introduction

Until 1930 the treatment of myasthenia gravis was "a source of discouragement to the patient and a cause of nightmare for the physician."[1] Bedrest for weeks or months was the most important therapeutic requisite, "with the hope that a remission may set in."[2] Slow spoon-feeding and diets high in calcium and albumin were also recommended, as well as tonics such as arsenic, phosphorus, quinine, iron or strychnine. Suprarenal, thymus, ovarian and testicular extracts sometimes improved and sometimes aggravated the symptoms, and radioactive thorium injections and roentgenotherapy to the thyroid and thymus were equally controversial.

However, accumulating knowledge about nitrogen-containing organic substances called "alkaloids," obtained from unrelated plants on three continents—the genus *Ephedra* from Asia, various curare-producing plants from South America, and *Physostigma venenosum* from Africa—would eventually converge to provide the first effective relief from the symptoms of myasthenia gravis. "Materia medica" was a very old term dating back to Dioscorides in the first century A.D., who used it to describe materials used to treat diseases.

Ma huang and Ephedrine

The Chinese herb *ma huang*, consisting of the stems from certain plants of the genus *Ephedra*, has been used by the Chinese for over 5,000 years to treat fevers and various other ailments. In 1885 **Nagayoshi Nagai**, Professor of Chemistry, and his Japanese colleagues at the University of Tokyo isolated and purified the active ingredient from *ma huang* and named this crystalline alkaloid "ephedrine."

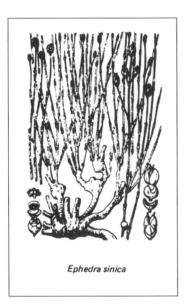

Ephedra sinica

EPHEDRA VULGARIS.—麻黄 (Ma-huang), 8or. **This** is a common plant in north China and Mongolia. The principal supply of the drug seems to have come from Honan province. The plant, with its leafless branches, has a slight resemblance to *Equisetum*, and in Japan as well as in China has been confounded with this latter. It bears yellow flowers, and produces red, edible berries, which have been likened to the raspberry. Pistillate and staminate flowers are borne on different plants. The drug consists of the yellow, jointed stems of the plant, tied up in bundles, or the stems from which the joints have been rejected, cut up into a chaff-like mass. The reason for rejecting the joints is because they are considered to have a medical action differing from, and in a measure counteracting that of the stems. The action is represented as decidedly diaphoretic and antipyretic. It is prescribed in fevers, especially malarial fever, in coughs, influenza, and post-partum difficulties. Its use should not be long continued, lest it weaken the body.

The root, which is also known as 狗骨 (Kou-ku), together with the joints, is considered to have an action directly opposed to that of the stem, and is therefore prescribed in profuse sweating, either critical or natural. It is used as a dusting powder, applied to the whole body. Although it probably has some astringent property, it is not recommended for any other difficulty, or to be used in any different way. The fruit is mucilaginous, with a slightly acrid or pungent flavor, and is eaten by the Chinese.

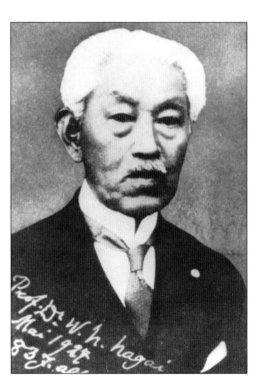

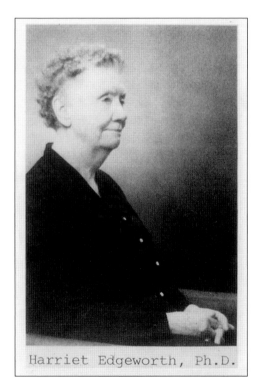

Harriet Edgeworth, Ph.D.

Ephedrine was introduced into Western medicine by **K.K. Chen** and **Carl F. Schmidt** in 1927. One of the persons who read about the re-isolation of ephedrine by Dr. Chen was **Harriet Edgeworth**, an American woman who had received her doctorate in chemistry from Columbia University and was in her fourth year at Rush Medical School when she came down with a severe case of myasthenia gravis. Because of its relationship to adrenaline she suggested to her doctors that ephedrine be tried for her myasthenia, but she was unable to convince them that it might be efficacious.

However, two years later, in 1929, Dr. Edgeworth noted immediate improvement of her myasthenia while taking a preparation of ephedrine and amidopyrine for menstrual cramps. Amidopyrine alone had no effect. She submitted a report of her personal experience with ephedrine to the *Journal of the American Medical Association* and it was published in April, 1930.[3] After three years of continued improvement, she published a confirmatory report in that same journal in 1933,[4] having established the optimal dose for her at 48 milligrams per day. She continued to take ephedrine for 18 years before it seemed to lose its effectiveness.

VOLUME 100
NUMBER 18

Clinical Notes, Suggestions and New Instruments

THE EFFECT OF EPHEDRINE IN THE TREATMENT OF
MYASTHENIA GRAVIS: SECOND REPORT

HARRIET EDGEWORTH, TUCSON, ARIZ.

Three years ago I[1] published a short report of progress on the use of ephedrine in a case of myasthenia gravis. The correspondence that has developed with physicians and relatives of patients having myasthenia gravis seems to make a further report desirable.

In the past three years, except for short periods when the ephedrine has been discontinued or the dose increased, for experimental purposes, I have taken a daily dose of ⅝ grain (48 mg.) of ephedrine sulphate or of ephedrine hydrochloride with slow but continuous improvement. The rate of improvement has been apparently uniform; that is, the amount of improvement during the last six months seems to have been as great as during the first six months. Larger doses give me a temporary increase in strength, but these dosages are invariably followed in two or three weeks by such adverse symptoms that I have always been compelled to reduce the dose. When in recent reports on the subject I see doses larger than those here recommended, I wonder how carefully and how long the effects of such dosages have been followed. The humiliating effect of helplessness leads both the myasthenic patient and his physician to seek the maximal effect from any remedy. This leads them to err on the side of excessive doses of ephedrine. In my experience, the dosage that will give the greatest effect in the first few weeks will not produce continuous and sustained improvement over a long period. An added advantage of using a smaller dose than the maximum that will be tolerated is that in emergencies, such as exposure to cold or heat, the depressing effects of a menstrual period, respiratory infections, or unusual exertion—all of which affect the myasthenic symptoms adversely—the dose can be temporarily increased with resulting benefit. As concrete examples of this, an extra dose of ephedrine before an unavoidable exposure to cold, as on a railroad or a motor trip, will prevent a severe stiffness in all my muscles which would otherwise occur and which would have such a temporary paralyzing effect that I would have to be lifted out of the car, or into the train.

Periods of intense heat are very prostrating to patients with myasthenia gravis; in fact, it may be the cause of death. For three summers I have definitely protected myself against this depressing effect by increasing the daily dose during a period of very hot weather. The myasthenic patient shows a progressive fatigue or weakness toward evening. However, the increased exertion that is possible on an increased dose is shown when I take an extra dose before going out to dinner in the evening. I am able to rise from the table unaided at the end of the dinner, behave as a normal person during the evening, and leave without falling down the front steps on departing. Without this extra dose I know from many embarrassing occasions that I should not be able to do this. A chronic sinus infection with recurring attacks which resisted all attempts at treatment locally disappeared after I began taking ephedrine. These recurring sinus infections so accelerated my downward progress that in 1927 I resorted to an autogenous vaccine, following which the sinus infections became less severe and less frequent, and there was some improvement in the myasthenic symptoms. But one week's use of ephedrine produced greater improvement than ten months' use of the vaccine. Although I live and associate normally with other people who occasionally have colds, I have been free from them for over two years.

The long continued use of ephedrine may produce adverse effects, the control of which I have begun to consider. But its beneficial effects far outweigh any of these I have discovered. As a matter of wisdom, I shall discontinue its use as soon as I can do so without losing the gains it has pro-

1. Edgeworth, Harriet: A Report of Progress on the Use of Ephedrine in a Case of Myasthenia Gravis, J. A. M. A. **94**:1136 (April 12).

Glycine

In her second paper Dr. Edgeworth referred to the work of **Walter M. Boothby** at the Mayo Clinic in Rochester, Minnesota. He published a series of papers between 1932 and 1936 in which he described the beneficial effects of the amino acid glycine (up to 30 milligrams per day) on the symptoms of myasthenia gravis.

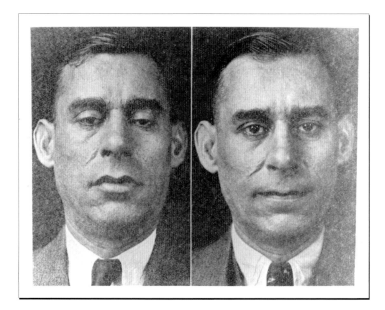

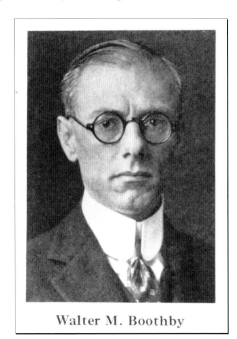

Walter M. Boothby

Pictured above is a before-and-after photograph[5] of a man with myasthenia gravis who returned to driving a truck while taking glycine, whereas before he had been barely able to walk. Although ephedrine is still used as a secondary medication in myasthenia, the reason for the disappearance of glycine from the medical armamentarium is unclear. The subsequent advent of "anti-curare" drugs may have lessened the enthusiasm for both ephedrine and glycine.

Curare

For centuries the indigenous people who live in the tropical forests of the headwaters of the Amazon River have tipped their hunting arrows with a tarry substance prepared from various plants. A good batch would completely paralyze a frog within one hop! Based on the type of container in which these preparations were stored, the material prepared from *Chondodendron* in the forest regions of Ecuador and Peru was called "tube-curare" by European travelers, whereas that derived from the creeping vine *Strychnos toxifera* in the more easterly regions in the Guianas and lower Orinoco was called "calabash-curare."

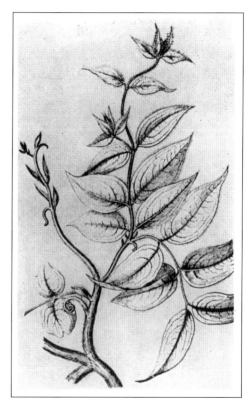

The liana, *Strychnos toxifera*, a source of curare.

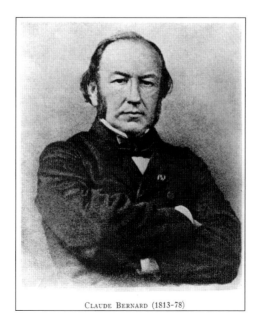

CLAUDE BERNARD (1813-78)

Although the native preparations of curare sent to Europe varied greatly in potency, in general calabash-curare was several hundred times more potent than tube-curare. **Claude Bernard**, the great French physiologist, used unpurified calabash-curare for his ingenious experiments with frogs, published between 1850 and 1857, described on page 34.

As illustrated, when a piece of curare was implanted (I) in the back of an intact frog, all the muscles became paralyzed except for those in one leg in which the circulation had been tied off; stimulation of the unligated sciatic nerve (N) continued to produce muscle twitches in that leg. Pinching the skin in the curare-poisoned regions also continued to produce reflex muscle contractions in the functional limb, suggesting to Bernard that the sensory nerves and central nervous system were not affected by curare. Stimulation of an isolated nerve placed in a bath containing curare (V) could still cause its muscle to contract, whereas a muscle (and the nerve endings) immersed in a bath containing curare (V') would no longer respond to stimulation of its nerve although it would continue to contract when stimulated directly. From these experiments Bernard reasoned that "curare must act on the terminal plates of motor nerves," even though the anatomy of the myoneural junction was still unclear at that time.[6]

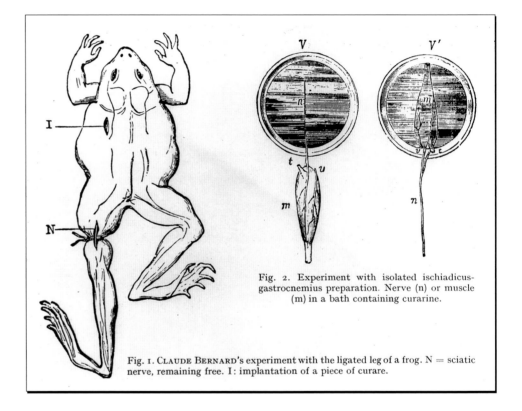

Fig. 2. Experiment with isolated ischiadicus-gastrocnemius preparation. Nerve (n) or muscle (m) in a bath containing curarine.

Fig. 1. CLAUDE BERNARD's experiment with the ligated leg of a frog. N = sciatic nerve, remaining free. I: implantation of a piece of curare.

Curare was often used by physiologists and pharmacologists in the 19th century to paralyze animals during their studies. At the turn of the century **J. Pal**, a pharmacologist in Vienna, was studying the action of physostigmine on the gut when he noticed that the paralysis of respiration induced by curare was removed by the injection of physostigmine, thus establishing that physostigmine is an antidote for curare.[7]

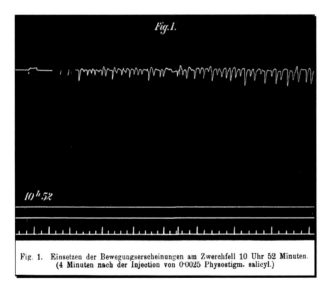 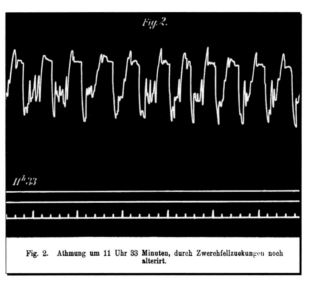 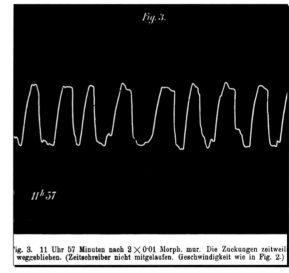

Fig. 1. Beginning of the motion of the diaphragm at 10 hours 52 minutes (4 minutes after the injection of 0.0025 Physostigmine salicylate).

Fig. 2. Respiration at 11 hours 33 minutes, altered by twitching of the diaphragm.

Fig. 3. At 11 hours 57 minutes after 2x0.01 morphine. The twitching disappears occasionally. (Time marks are not present. Same speed as in Fig. 2.)

Physosigmine

Physostigmine is the active ingredient of the Calabar bean, a dried ripe seed of *Physostigma venenosum*, a perennial woody climber growing on the banks of streams in tropical West Africa. The "ordeal bean" was a ritual used by the indigenous rulers to determine the guilt or innocence of those who were forced to swallow it. Presumably the innocent swallowed it whole and promptly vomited it up, while the guilty nibbled bits of it, absorbed them, and died![7]

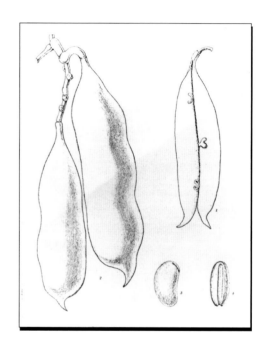

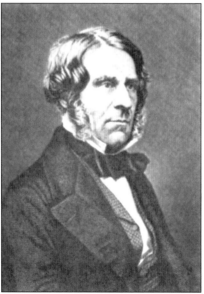

Robert Christison

Calabar beans, brought from West Africa to Scotland by Presbyterian missionaries, were planted and cultivated in botanical gardens there. In 1855 **Robert Christison**, Professor of Materia Medica and Therapeutics at the University of Edinburgh, survived his own ordeal after intentionally ingesting one-quarter of a Calabar bean.

Christison's pupil and successor, **Thomas Richard Fraser**, isolated an amorphous active principle from the kernel of the Calabar bean in 1863 and proposed to call it "eserine" after the name for the ordeal poison in Calabar. In 1864 it was isolated in completely pure form in Germany and called "physostigmine," whereas in 1865 it was obtained in crystalline form in France and named "eserine." Both names are still used.

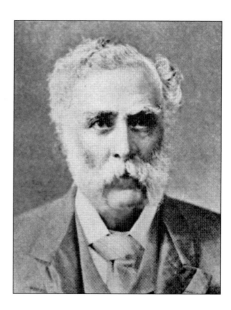

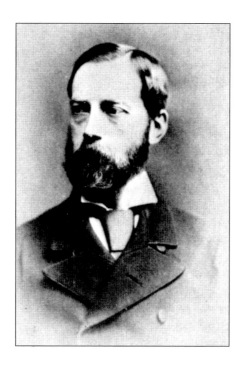

On a hint from Fraser, **Douglas Moray Cooper Lamb Argyll Robertson** used an extract of the Calabar bean as a young man in 1863 to stimulate the pupillary sphincter of the eye, counteracting the dilating action of atropine.

Mary Broadfoot Walker

Women were not admitted to the University of Edinburgh when **Mary Broadfoot Walker** graduated from the Glasgow & Edinburgh Medical College for Women in 1913. She was therefore probably unaware of the important association of Scotland with physostigmine when as a junior house officer at St. Alfege's Hospital in Greenwich, a suburb of London, she became the first to try physostigmine as a treatment for myasthenia gravis. Apparently she was prompted to try this drug because of an analogy her neurology consultant, **Derek Denny-Brown**, made between myasthenia gravis and curare poisoning.[8]

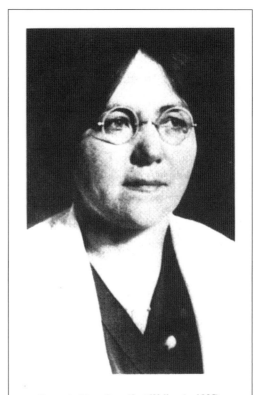

Figure 1. Mary Broadfoot Walker (c. 1935).

In a brief letter[9] submitted to the medical journal Lancet on May 12, 1934 – the same day that **Sir Henry Dale** and **W. Feldberg** presented to a meeting of the Physiological Society the first experimental evidence for a possible role of acetylcholine at the neuromuscular junction – Mary Walker described the temporary improvement in eyelid strength, jaw strength, arm strength and swallowing of a 56-year-old woman with MG following the subcutaneous injection of physostigmine sulfate, grain 1/60 (0.5 mg).

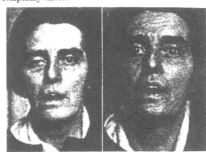

1200 THE LANCET] TREATMENT OF MYASTHENIA GRAVIS WITH PHYSOSTIGMINE [JUNE 2, 1934

CORRESPONDENCE

TREATMENT OF MYASTHENIA GRAVIS WITH PHYSOSTIGMINE

To the Editor of THE LANCET

SIR,—The abnormal fatiguability in myasthenia gravis has been thought to be due to curare-like poisoning of the motor nerve-endings or of the "myoneural junctions" in the affected muscles. It occurred to me recently that it would be worth while to try the effect of physostigmine, a partial antagonist to curare, on a case of myasthenia gravis at present in St. Alfege's Hospital, in the hope that it would counteract the effect of the unknown substance which might be exerting a curare-like effect on the myoneural junctions. I found that hypodermic injections of physostigmine salicylate did have a striking though temporary effect.

I think that this effect of physostigmine on myasthenia gravis is important, though it is only temporary, for it improves swallowing and might tide a patient over a respiratory crisis. It supports the opinion that the fatiguability is due to a poisoning of the motor end-organs, or "myoneural junctions," rather than to an affection of the muscle itself. It may be significant that physostigmine inhibits the action of the esterase which destroys acetylcholine. I have not had the opportunity of treating another case to confirm the findings. The administration of other drugs whose action resembles that of physostigmine is under consideration. It is also possible that physostigmine might be of some service in botulism and in cobra poisoning, in both of which a curare-like poisoning of the "myoneural junctions" of the respiratory muscles has been stated to be the main cause of death.

I wish to thank Dr. Philip Hamill for his interest and advice, and Dr. W. D. Wiggins, medical superintendent of the hospital, for permission to publish the case.   I am, Sir, yours faithfully,
M. B. WALKER.

St. Alfege's Hospital, Greenwich, May 12th.

Before injection the patient cannot raise her left eyelid. Thirty minutes after it the eye is fully open. (The photographs are reproduced from a cinematograph film and are reversed left for right.)

Prostigmin

Two weeks after her physostigmine letter had been published in *Lancet*, Mary Walker successfully treated another MG patient with neostigmine methylsulfate, a proprietary analogue of physostigmine named "Prostigmin" by Roche Laboratories in Basel, Switzerland. She noted that the advantages of Prostigmin over physostigmine were its relative safety and less potential for side effects, but the disadvantage was its expense, "the price of an ampoule containing 0.5 mg of the drug being ninepence." She demonstrated the rapid effect of Prostigmin at a meeting of the Clinical Section of the Royal Society of Medicine on February 8, 1935.[10]

Case showing the Effect of Prostigmin on Myasthenia Gravis.—M. B. WALKER, M.R.C.P.

D. C., female, aged 40.

History.—In spring 1930 she noticed undue fatigability of the arms and drooping of the right upper eyelid. In July 1930 she was admitted to the Middlesex Hospital with diplopia, and was discharged, appreciably better, within a month. January 1931, readmitted with impairment of all movements of the left eye and weakness of the arms and legs, which became worse towards the end of the day. In

April she had difficulty in swallowing and regurgitation of fluids through the nose. She was treated with ephedrine with improvement, and whenever the ephedrine was stopped the symptoms became worse. She was at work from September 1931 to September 1933, taking ephedrine all the time. In May 1933 she again complained of diplopia, and in September she was readmitted to the Middlesex Hospital where she was treated with glycine and ephedrine, but did not respond so well. No ephedrine was given after she left the Middlesex Hospital.

In September 1934 the symptoms became worse and she was transferred to St. Alfege's Hospital on October 24.

Condition on admission.—Ptosis of left upper eyelid; partial external ophthalmoplegia; weakness of arms, especially of flexors of fingers; weakness of muscles of back, and of lower limbs. The thyroid was enlarged, but the thymus was not.

She had great difficulty in raising herself up in bed, could only walk a few yards unsteadily, could not feed herself after the first few mouthfuls, and complained of diplopia. Speech was slow and became indistinct after a few sentences. Swallowing was difficult and fluids regurgitated through the nose.

Her condition has remained unchanged except that she has not complained of diplopia for the last few days, and her grip is stronger than it was on admission.

A hypodermic injection of prostigmin relieves these symptoms temporarily. Atropine given at the same time prevents colic and nausea without affecting the action of prostigmin on the motor nerve-endings.

Since December 18, 1934, she has had 2·5 mgm. of prostigmin and 0·66 mgm. of atropine daily at 10 a.m. Five minutes after the injection the ptosis and external ophthalmoplegia disappear, a few minutes later she sits up in bed easily, in ten to fifteen minutes she can walk several hundred yards without feeling tired. After the effect of the injection on the fatigability has worn off, the muscles feel a little stiff.

The effect is at its height an hour after the injection and begins to wear off gradually in about six hours. Occasionally a second injection is given at 4 p.m. and the effect lasts until late in the evening.

Smaller injections were given at first, with the following results:—

Amount of prostigmin Mgm.		Onset of effect (Minutes)		Duration of effect (Hours)
0·5	...	30-45	...	2·3
1·0	...	20	...	4·5
1·5	...	10	...	4·5
2·0	...	8	...	5·6
2·5	...	5	...	6·8

The larger the dose, the greater the increase of muscular power.

Given by the mouth 1·5 mgm. of prostigmin caused nausea, the effect was much less, and came on much later than when the drug was given hypodermically.

Control injections of ephedrine, lobeline, femergin, and water produced no effect on the muscular weakness.

Physostigmine salicylate, 1 mgm. approximately, removed the ptosis but made the patient feel sick and faint and disinclined to move. Atropine given with the physostigmine counteracts these ill-effects, without altering the action on the motor nerve-endings.

Physostigmine salicylate was given in a previous case of the disease which was admitted to St. Alfege's Hospital in April 1934, because it was thought that as the muscles in myasthenia gravis behave like muscles poisoned by curare, physostigmine, an antagonist to curare, might also counteract the unknown substance which might be exerting a curare-like effect on the motor nerve-endings in myasthenia gravis. The patient tolerated it well, and its effect on the weakness and fatigability was the same as that of prostigmin, 1·0 mgm.

The advantages of prostigmin (Roche)—a synthetic drug analogous to physostigmine and with similar actions—over physostigmine are that it has a less depressing effect on the heart, less often causes nausea and vomiting, and is probably safer in large doses; 4 mgm. have been given without ill-effect, though in other cases the same dose has caused severe diarrhœa and cardiac and respiratory distress. The disadvantage is its expense, the price of an ampoule containing 0·5 mgm. of the drug, being ninepence.

Dr. P. HAMILL: Whatever may be the mechanism of the weakness and fatigability of the muscles in myasthenia gravis, physostigmine, and its ally, prostigmin, overcome it. The resulting voluntary movements are normal in type. If it is the case that nervous impulses set free acetylcholine—or some analogous substance at the nerve-endings, and that in myasthenia the supply is deficient, physostigmine, by delaying its destruction, would compensate for the lack.

On this hypothesis, defective innervation, whether resulting from some disability of the anterior-horn cells or impaired conduction of nerve-fibres, as in neuritis, should also be corrected by injection of physostigmine and prostigmin. This appears to be the case, the drugs having been used in cases of peripheral neuritis and in spinal-cord lesions with beneficial results. Muscular power is increased. As additions to massage in such cases, the drugs may help in maintaining nutrition of the paralysed muscles and thus accelerate their recovery. The economic aspects are important. A wide field of usefulness in neuro-muscular disorders is thus opened and is now being studied; the results will be communicated at a later date.

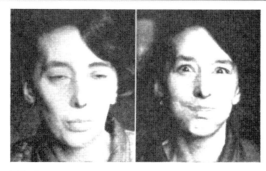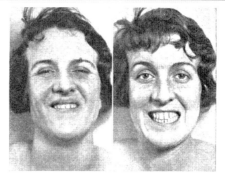

FIG. 1 (CASE 1).—In each of these photographs the patient is making her maximal effort to distend the cheeks with air. Before injection of prostigmin (left) the weakness of the lip musculature did not allow any detectable inflation of the cheeks. The improvement after injection is seen on the right.

FIG. 2 (CASE 5).—In these photographs the patient is making a maximal effort to show her teeth with the jaws shut. The weakness of the retractors and the substitution of the elevators of the upper lip is seen in the left-hand photograph, taken before injection of prostigmin. The increased power of the retractors after injection is seen on the right.

E. A. Blake Pritchard, *Lancet*, February 23, 1935.

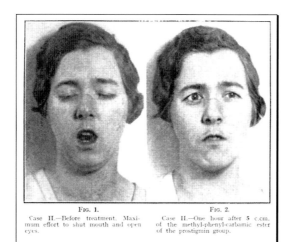

FIG. 1.
Case II.—Before treatment. Maximum effort to shut mouth and open eyes.

FIG. 2.
Case II.—One hour after 5 c.cm. of the methyl-phenyl-carbamic ester of the prostigmin group.

L. P. E. Laurent, *British Medical Journal*, March 9, 1935.

Beneficial effects of Prostigmin were quickly confirmed by physicians from University College, London.[11, 12]

Mary Walker, with her brief case reports and her frequent demonstrations, not only offered symptomatic treatment for MG that has stood the test of time, but also provided the most convincing evidence at the time that the neuromuscular junction was the focus of the disease.

References for Chapter 3: From Plants to Materia Medica (1927-1935)

1. Kennedy FS, Moersch FP: Myasthenia gravis: A clinical review of eighty-seven cases observed between 1915 and the early part of 1932. *Canadian Medical Association J* 37:216-223, 1935.

2. Keschner M, Strauss I: Myasthenia gravis. *Archives of Neurology and Psychiatry* 17:337-376, 1927.

3. Edgeworth H: A report of progress on the use of ephedrine in a case of myasthenia gravis. *J American Medical Association* 94:1136, 1930.

4. Edgeworth H: The effect of ephedrine in the treatment of myasthenia gravis: Second report. *J American Medical Association* 100:1401, 1933.

5. Boothby WM: Second report on the effect of treatment with glycine. *Proceedings of the Staff Meetings of the Mayo Clinic* 7:737-742, 1932.

6. Bernard C: *Leçons sur les effect des substances toxiques et médicamenteuses*, Paris, pp. 238-353, 1857.

7. Pal J: Physostigmin ein Gegengift des Curare. *Zentralblatt Physiologische* 14:255-258, 1900, cited in B Holmstedt, "The ordeal bean of Old Calabar: The pageant of *Physostigma venenosum* in medicine," in T Swain (editor), *Plants in the development of modern medicine.* Harvard University Press, Cambridge, 1972.

8. Keesey J: Contemporary opinions about Mary Walker, a shy pioneer of therapeutic neurology. *Neurology* 51:1433-1439, 1998.

9. Walker MB: Treatment of myasthenia gravis with physostigmine. *Lancet* 1:1200-1201, 1934.

10. Walker MB: Case showing the effect of Prostigmin on myasthenia gravis. *Proceedings of the Royal Society of Medicine* 28:759-761, 1935.

11. Laurent LPE: Clinical observations of the use of Prostigmin in the treatment of myasthenia gravis. *British Medical J* 1:463-465, 1935.

12. Pritchard EAB: The use of "Prostigmin" in treatment of myasthenia gravis. *Lancet* 1:432-435, 1935.

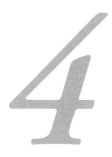

Thymectomy and the Autoimmune Hypothesis (1936-1960)

Introduction

As described in Chapter 2, thymic tumors were often found post-mortem in patients who died with myasthenia gravis. However, before such tumors in the chest could be removed during life, some way had to be devised of keeping the lungs inflated when the chest was opened. Normally the moist outer lining of the lungs adheres to the moist inner lining of the chest wall, but if atmospheric pressure is allowed to penetrate these linings, the lungs collapse.

From the 18th century on, various mechanical methods were devised to inflate the collapsed lungs via the mouth or windpipe using pipes, bellows or bags, a method now called "positive pressure ventilation." Even as late as the 1952 poliomyelitis epidemic in Scandinavia, scores of medical students took turns ventilating polio victims by manually squeezing a rubber bag connected to the patient's airway! Eventually machines were developed to perform this task automatically, and since the 1960's mechanical positive pressure ventilation in intensive care units has greatly improved the survival of patients with myasthenia gravis whose breathing becomes impaired.

A second method, called "negative pressure ventilation" in which sub-atmospheric pressure was intermittently developed around the thorax and abdomen, was also used to assist respiration. The most famous of these negative pressure ventilators, and the first to be of long-term clinical value, was the "iron lung," developed in 1929 by **Philip Drinker**, an engineer at Harvard Medical School. For surgery of the chest, however, a large negative pressure chamber was conceived by the famous Professor of Surgery at the University of Zurich in Switzerland, **Ernst Ferdinand Sauerbruch**.

Sauerbruch was the surgeon who, in March, 1911, first successfully removed the thymus in a patient with myasthenia gravis.[1] An enlarged thymus was visible on radiographs of a 20-year-old woman with both MG and hyperthyroidism. At that time partial thymectomy (thymus reduction) was a treatment for hyperthyroidism. Sauerbruch removed the patient's thymus through an incision in the neck, thereby avoiding the necessity of using his cumbersome low-pressure chamber. Her doctors were surprised that after surgery there was more improvement of the patient's myasthenic symptoms than of the symptoms of hyperthyroidism. Subsequently Sauerbruch treated the latter by also removing the patient's thyroid.

In the 1930's, Sauerbruch removed a large thymoma from each of two patients with myasthenia gravis, but both patients died from infection a few days post-operatively. In a review in 1936, Lièvre stated that there existed no published report of the successful removal of a thymoma during life.

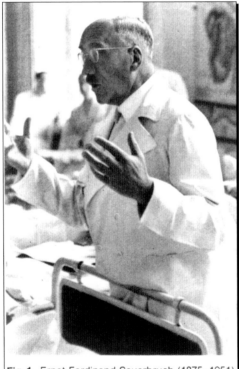

Fig. 1. Ernst Ferdinand Sauerbruch (1875–1951)

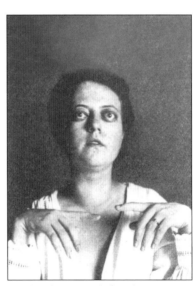

Sauerbruch's patient before the operation

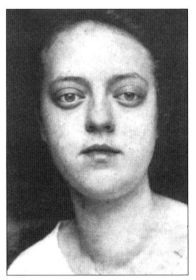

Same patient post-operatively

In the same year that Lièvre wrote that no thymoma had ever been removed successfully, the American surgeon **Alfred Blalock** at Vanderbilt University in Nashville, Tennessee, removed the cystic remains of a necrotic thymic tumor which had previously been treated by two courses of thymic radiation. Reported in 1939,[2] Blalock used intra-tracheal intubation, positive pressure ventilation and a midline sternal approach. The 21-year-old patient had had generalized myasthenia for four years prior to surgery. Within three years after surgery she obtained complete remission and was still in good health 21 years later.

Two and a half weeks after he assumed the Chair of Surgery at Johns Hopkins University School of Medicine on July 1, 1941, Blalock performed the first transsternal thymectomy for a patient with myasthenia who did not have a thymoma. Encouraged by Johns Hopkins physicians **A. McGehee Harvey, Frank Ford,** and **Joseph Lilienthal**, Blalock successfully performed six such operations during the next six weeks. Only four months after the first operation, on November 1, 1941, a preliminary report of these cases was published in the *Journal of the American Medical Association* claiming improvement had resulted in most of the cases.[3]

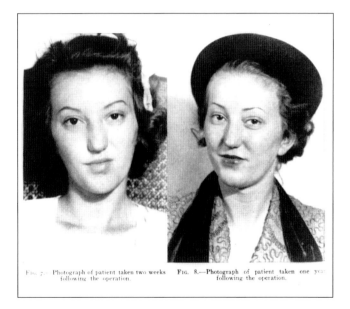

FIG. 7.—Photograph of patient taken two weeks following the operation.   FIG. 8.—Photograph of patient taken one year following the operation.

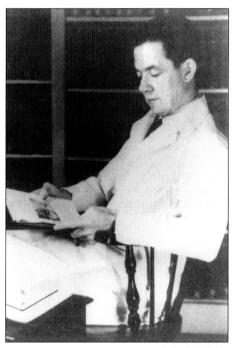

Alfred Blalock

Controversy about Thymectomy for Myasthenia Gravis, 1949-1953

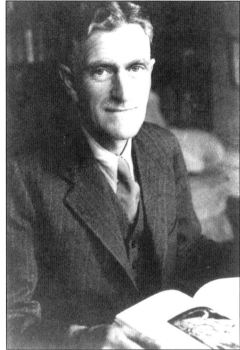

Sir Geoffrey Keynes

In London the surgeon **Geoffrey Keynes** was stimulated by Blalock's preliminary report. He performed the first thymectomy for myasthenia gravis in England on February 10, 1942, on a 31-year-old woman with severe and progressive disease who then "went on to lead a productive life." By 1949 Keynes had operated on 155 myasthenic patients, 120 of whom did not have tumors. He claimed that 65% of the non-tumorous group had shown a complete or almost complete remission of symptoms.[5] However, his tumor cases did so poorly that Keynes concluded that the presence of a thymoma was a contraindication to surgery.

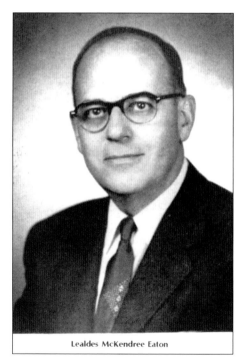

Lealdes McKendree Eaton

The Mayo Clinic in Rochester, Minnesota, disagreed with Keynes about the beneficial effect of thymectomy. **Lee Eaton**, the neurologist, and **O. Theron Clagett**, the surgeon from the Mayo Clinic, reported in the *Journal of the American Medical Association* in 1950 on 72 thymectomies for MG compared to 142 non-surgical MG "controls." They concluded that there was *"no indication that thymectomy influences beneficially the course of myasthenia gravis. This opinion is reached in spite of the fact that in several cases recovery following thymectomy has been dramatic."*[6]

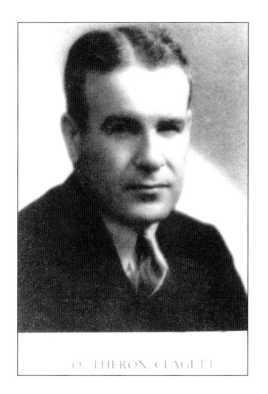

O. THERON CLAGETT

Keynes, feeling discredited, as he put it, "with douches of cold water drawn from the Mayo Clinic cistern," experienced widespread criticism but realized that while he had reported his surgical results separately on patients with tumors and those without tumors, the Mayo Clinic had lumped the results of the two groups together to reach their opposite conclusion.[7] When forced to recalculate their results after separating patients with and without tumors, Eaton and Clagett reported in an obscure journal[8] that 50% of the surgical group without tumors had a good result, over twice that of the non-surgical group without tumors, *"thereby justifying the expense, discomfort and risk of surgery."*

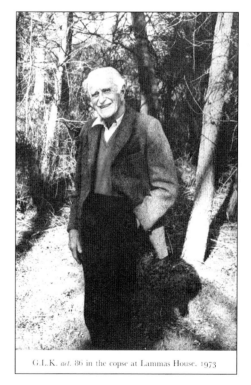

G.L.K. *aet.* 86 in the copse at Lammas House. 1973

The controversy about the results of thymectomy continues to this day, but this cautionary tale of clinical research from the 1950's is still worth remembering. Keynes, the brother of the economist John Maynard Keynes and an esteemed bibliographer of Donne and Blake, was knighted in 1955 and at age 94 published a delightful autobiography of his eventful life.[9]

Simpson: Clinical Clues to Autoimmunity in Myasthenia Gravis, 1958-1960

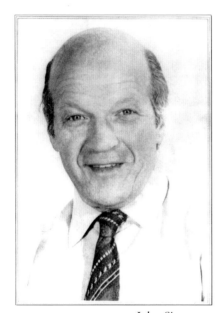

John Simpson

This trans-Atlantic disagreement about thymectomy eventually led to an important development in our understanding of myasthenia. The Scottish physician **John Simpson**, while on a Medical Research Council Fellowship at The National Hospital, Queen Square, London, was asked by **Dr. Arnold Carmichael** to evaluate all the patients with myasthenia gravis seen at The National Hospital since 1934. Keynes invited Simpson to include also in the analysis all the myasthenic patients operated on by Keynes at New End and St. Bartholomew's Hospitals as well. From this evaluation of 404 MG patients,[10] Simpson concluded that there was a substantial chance of improvement after thymectomy, especially early in the disease if no thymoma was present.

AN EVALUATION OF
THYMECTOMY IN MYASTHENIA GRAVIS

BY

JOHN A. SIMPSON[1]

(*From The Neurological Research Unit of the Medical Research Council,
The National Hospital, Queen Square, London*)

BRAIN 81: 112 (1958)

John A. Simpson

Neurology Unit of the University Department of Medicine, Northern General Hospital, Edinburgh

TABLE XXV.—COMPARISON OF NON-TUMOUR CASES WITH OTHER SERIES

| Series* | | Operated | | | | Not-operated | | | |
		London %	Mayo %	Boston %	Balti- more %	London %	Mayo %	Boston %	Balti- more %
A	F	22·0	16·7	20·7	12·0	15·3	5·6	13·0	14·0
B		13·2	36·7	41·5	36·0	5·1	14·8	20·7	22·0
C		23·1	20·0			15·3	14·8		
D		17·6	16·7	22·6	24·0	13·5	57·4	37·7	34·0
Data incomplete		7·1	—	—	—	15·3			
Myasth. deaths		7·7	6·6	7·6		28·8	7·4	28·3..	30·0
Post-op. deaths		7·7 ⎱17·0	6·3	7·5	28·0	— ⎱35·6			
Deaths, other		1·6	—	—		6·8			
	Total cases	182	30	53	25	59	54	53	77
A	M	19·7	17·7	8·0	22·0	17·5	13·0	16·0	17·0
B		10·5	17·7	16·0	16·0	5·0	17·4	10·0	12·0
C		23·7	17·7			7·5	17·4		
D		19·7	35·3	44·0	21·0	25·0	43·5	24·0	27·0
Data incomplete		5·3	—	—	—	22·5	—		
Myasth. deaths		11·8	0	8·0		20·0	8·7	20·0	
Post-op. deaths		7·9 ⎱21·0	11·8	24·0	42·0	— ⎱22·5	—	—	44·0
Deaths, others		1·3	—	—		2·5			
	Total cases	76	17	25	19	40	23	25	41

*London—present series. Mayo Clinic—Eaton and Clagett (1955). Boston—Schwab and Leland (1953). Baltimore—Grob (1953).

The Journal of the Royal Medico-Chirurgical Society of Glasgow, the Medico-Chirurgical
Society of Edinburgh, and the Edinburgh Obstetrical Society

Volume 5 OCTOBER 1960 Number 10

SCOTTISH MEDICAL JOURNAL

MYASTHENIA GRAVIS: A NEW HYPOTHESIS*

John A. Simpson

Neurology Unit of the University Department of Medicine, Northern General Hospital, Edinburgh

IN a part of the world which has now adopted more sophisticated methods of brain washing, it was once the custom to expose those with unorthodox ideas to a trial by ordeal which consisted of the chewing of the Calabar bean. Today I wish to present you with some unorthodox ideas so let me start by asking you to throw away the Calabar bean, or at least to keep its active constituent, physostigmine, out of sight, for I believe that this magic bean, or its synthetic competitors may have blurred our vision of the true nature of myasthenia gravis.

First let me pay tribute to Mrs Honyman-Gillespie who has made these lectures possible and the Post-Graduate Committee who invited me to contribute to this famous series. The first lecture was given by Edwin Bramwell (1938) on the contributions of the Edinburgh school to the study of the reactions of the pupil of the eye. From him I learned that the mydriatic action of the Calabar bean was discovered by Sir Thomas Fraser in 1863 when he was professor of materia medica in Edinburgh and a physician to the Royal Infirmary, and introduced to ophthalmological practice in the same year by the young Argyll Robertson in a paper read before the Medico-Chirurgical Society of Edinburgh.

Collier (1930) attributed the first British *recognition* of myasthenia gravis to this same Edwin Bramwell when he was starting his illustrious neurological career as a house-physician at Queen Square. Though first described by the Englishman Thomas Willis in 1672, the syndrome was unrecognized until the magnificent papers of Erb (1879) and

Goldflam (1893). Indeed, Bramwell's father, Byrom Bramwell, gives an excellent description of a case in his famous *Atlas* (1892a) but could not name it, and the illustration reproduced in Figure 1 is almost certainly a myasthenic child. Edwin Bramwell with Campbell reviewed the known cases in 1900 (Campbell & Bramwell, 1900) and recognition became more common from that time on. If some of the facts I shall present are unfamiliar it is humbling to record that almost all are present in that instructive review or in the interesting paper by their colleague Buzzard (1905). They have been ignored, and many later observations discarded because they are difficult to reconcile with views which have been current since attention was focussed on the phenomena of neuromuscular transmission which is presumed to be disturbed in myasthenia gravis.

I would like you to forget all that you have been taught or presumed with regard to myasthenia and look with me at the symptoms and signs present in a series of 440 cases which I have been privileged to examine through the kindness of colleagues in Edinburgh, London and Glasgow. Let us not decide what is 'relevant' until the whole picture is before us. I shall draw some novel conclusions from this analysis, leading to a new hypothesis. This will probably require modification in detail but has the double merit of incorporating all the clinical phenomena without exception, and of suggesting completely new lines of inquiry. In the closing part of the lecture a necessarily brief account of the pathophysiology and pharmacology of myasthenia will be given to demonstrate that the hypothesis is compatible with the known facts.

*A Honyman-Gillespie Lecture delivered on 28th April 1960.

During his survey of these 404 patients, Simpson recorded that myasthenia gravis was associated not only with thyrotoxicosis (hyperthyroidism) but with other thyroid diseases, as well as with rheumatoid arthritis, "diffuse" lupus erythematosis, sarcoidosis, and reticuloendothelial disorders resembling lupus erythematosus. He was impressed by the similarities between myasthenia and lupus in age, sex and fluctuating symptoms, and he also noticed a high incidence of thyrotoxicosis in close relatives of myasthenics. Although none of these conditions, except thyroiditis, was known to be autoimmune at that time, Simpson thought that these associations, as well as the thymic abnormalities and muscle lymphorrhages in myasthenia, suggested an immune process. He credited **D. W. Smithers** with the first suggestion (during a speech on thyroid tumors in 1958) that myasthenia like thyroiditis *"may also be due to an auto-immune response associated at times with neoplasia."* Simpson hypothesized in 1960 that myasthenia gravis was *"an 'auto-immune' response of muscle in which an antibody to endplate protein may be formed,"*[11] perhaps a response to an infection or the reaction of the thymus under the influence of the pituitary gland.

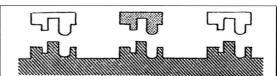

Fig. 16. Two molecules of acetylcholine and one of antibody have similar configuration, based on endplate receptor 'templates'. They will compete for receptor sites.

Early Laboratory Evidence for Autoimmunity in Myasthenia Gravis, 1954-1963

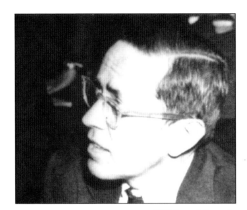

William Nastuk

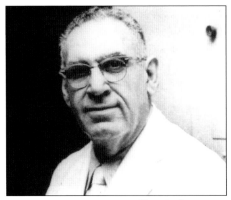

Kermit Osserman

Although early authors as far back as 1900 had speculated that a toxic agent circulating in the blood might be responsible for the fluctuating symptoms of myasthenia gravis, the demonstration by Mary Walker in 1938 of increased ptosis when a tourniquet around an exercised limb was released gave impetus to the search for a circulating factor in MG.

In 1954 **William Nastuk**, a physiologist working on basic aspects of neuromuscular transmission at Columbia University in New York City, was approached by **Arthur Strauss**, a medical student in the College of Physicians and Surgeons at Columbia, about re-examining the circulating factor hypothesis. Nastuk began to perfuse frog nerve-muscle preparations with dilutions of sera from MG patients, collected for him by **Kermit Osserman**, the director of the large Myasthenia Gravis Clinic at Mount Sinai Hospital in New York City. Some of these sera produced a moth-eaten appearance of superficial frog muscle fibers, suggesting the possibility of an antigen-antibody reaction with serum "complement," an array of serum proteins that bind with antigen-antibody complexes to destroy cell surfaces. Nastuk therefore collaborated with **Otto Plescia**, who was studying complement in the Department of Microbiology at Columbia, on serial complement levels in patients with myasthenia. They found that these serum complement levels fell during clinical exacerbations of myasthenia and were higher during remissions, suggesting to them *"the possibility that an immune mechanism may play an etiological role in myasthenia gravis."* This work was published by Nastuk, Osserman and Plescia in abstract form in 1956[12] and in more detail in 1960.[13]

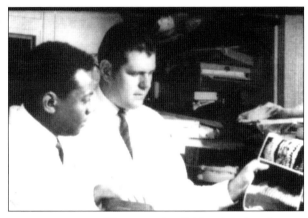
Hugo van der Geld and Arthur Strauss

Meanwhile, after graduating from medical school in 1958 and finishing his internship at Mount Sinai Hospital, **Arthur Strauss** began studying the possibility of cross-reactivity between chick striated muscle and chick thymus using the fluorescent antibody technique of **Drs. Beatrice Seegal** and **Konrad Hsu** in the Department of Microbiology at Columbia. In 1960 Strauss demonstrated that some pooled myasthenic sera, particularly those of patients with thymomas, contained complement-fixing globulins (antibodies?) which, if tagged with a fluorescent dye marker, produced an alternating staining pattern under the ultraviolet microscope corresponding to the micro-anatomical structure of striated muscle.[14] Strauss continued this work as an investigator at the National Institute of Allergy and Infectious Diseases at the National Institutes of Health in Bethesda, Maryland. He was joined there by **Hugo van der Geld**, a Surinamese-born Dutch-trained cardiologist who in 1963 with **Hans Oosterhuis** in Amsterdam had found large cells in calf thymus, perhaps the myoid cells described in Chapter 2 (page 23), which were also similarly stained with MG sera.[15] This provided the first clue connecting a disorder of neuromuscular transmission with thymus abnormalities.

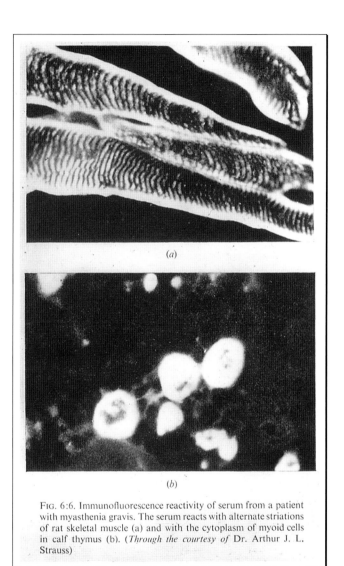

(a)

(b)

FIG. 6:6. Immunofluorescence reactivity of serum from a patient with myasthenia gravis. The serum reacts with alternate striations of rat skeletal muscle (a) and with the cytoplasm of myoid cells in calf thymus (b). (*Through the courtesy of* Dr. Arthur J. L. Strauss)

S impson's hypothesis and the back-to-back papers by Nastuk and Strauss all appeared in October 1960. In 1960 the role of the thymus was still unknown, and although it seemed to play some role in myasthenia gravis, immunologists considered it *"a vestigial structure filled with incompetent cells and a graveyard for dying lymphocytes,"* according to **Jacques F. A. P. Miller** of the Walter and Eliza Hall Institute of Medical Research in Victoria, Australia. As a result of his Ph.D. work at the Chester Beatty Research Institute near London on leukemic neoplasms, Miller published in *Lancet* in 1961 a preliminary report of the results of his experiments on thymectomized newborn mice which demonstrated that the thymus had an important role in the maturation of lymphocytes, which then migrated to other sites in the body at about the time of birth.[16] This was the beginning of the recognition of the immunological function of lymphocytes and of the importance of the thymus in immune processes. Back in Australia, Miller later went on to demonstrate the difference between thymus-derived and bone-marrow derived lymphocytes.

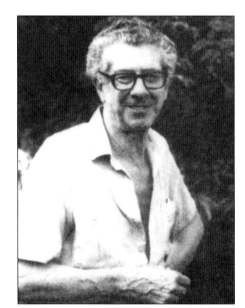

Jacques F.A.P. Miller at Cold
Springs Harbor, 1989

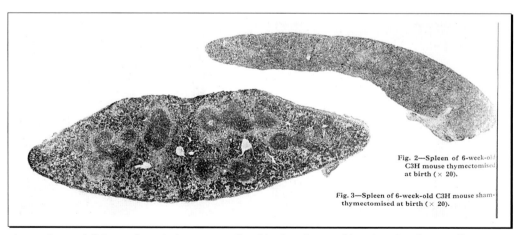

Fig. 2—Spleen of 6-week-old C3H mouse thymectomised at birth (× 20).

Fig. 3—Spleen of 6-week-old C3H mouse sham-thymectomised at birth (× 20).

A conspicuous deficiency of germinal centers was found in the spleens and lymph nodes of neonatally thymectomized mice.

References for Chapter 4: Thymectomy and the Autoimmune Hypothesis (1936-1960)

1. Schumacher CH, Roth, P: Thymektomie bei einem Fall von Murbus Basedowi mit Myasthenia. *Mitteilungen aus den Grenzgebeiten der Medizin und Chirurgie* 25:746-765, 1913.

2. Blalock A, Mason MF, Morgan HJ, Riven SS: Myasthenia gravis and tumors of the thymic region. Report of a case in which the tumor was removed. *Annals of Surgery* 110:544-559, 1939.

3. Blalock A, Harvey AM, Ford FF, Lilienthal JL: The treatment of myasthenia gravis by removal of the thymus gland. *J American Medical Association* 117:1529-1533, 1941.

4. Blalock A: in Discussion, p. 78, of Clagett OT, Eaton LM. Surgical treatment of myasthenia gravis. *J Thoracic Surgery* 16:62-80, 1947.

5. Keynes G: The results of thymectomy in myasthenia gravis. *British Medical J* 1:611-616. 1949.

6. Eaton LM, Clagett OT: Thymectomy in the treatment of myasthenia gravis. *J American Medical Association* 142:963-967, 1950.

7. Keynes G: Surgery of the thymus gland, second (and third) thoughts. *Lancet* 1:1197-1201, 1954.

8. Eaton LM, Clagett OT, Bastron JA: Chapter V: The thymus and its relationship to diseases of the nervous system; Study of 374 cases of myasthenia gravis and comparison of 87 patients undergoing thymectomy with 225 controls. *Proceedings of the Association for Research on Nervous & Mental Diseases* 32:107-124, 1953.

9. Keynes G: *The Gates of Memory.* Clarendon Press, Oxford, 1981.

10. Simpson J: An evaluation of thymectomy in myasthenia gravis. *Brain* 81:112-144, 1958.

11. Simpson J: Myasthenia gravis: A new hypothesis. *Scottish Medical J* 5:419-436, 1960.

12. Nastuk WL, Osserman KE, Plescia OJ: Reduction in serum complement concentration in myasthenia gravis. *Federation Proceedings* 15:135-136, 1956.

13. Nastuk WL, Plescia OJ, Osserman KE: Changes in serum complement activity in patients with myasthenia gravis. *Proceedings of the Society for Experimental Biology & Medicine* 105:177-184, 1960.

14. Strauss AJL, Seegal BC, Hsu KC, Burkholder PM, Nastuk WL, Osserman KE: Immunofluorescence demonstration of a muscle binding, complement fixing serum globulin fraction in myasthenia gravis. *Proceedings of the Society for Experimental Biology & Medicine* 105:184-191, 1960.

15. van der Geld H, Oosterhuis HJGH: Muscle and thymus antibodies in myasthenia gravis. *Vox Sanguinis* 8:196-204, 1963.

16. Miller JFAP: Immunological function of the thymus. *Lancet* 2:748-749, 1961.

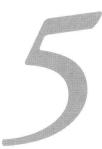

Presynaptic, Synaptic or Postsynaptic? (1935-1977)

Introduction

Despite the growing body of information about thymic abnormalities, muscle lymphorrhages, autoimmunity and various medication benefits that have been reviewed in previous chapters, the reason why patients with myasthenia become weak still remained a mystery. The improvement with "Prostigmin" suggested that some abnormality of the myoneural junction was most likely, but there was considerable disagreement for decades about whether the site of the problem was on the nerve side (presynaptic), the muscle side (post-synaptic) or in between (synaptic). Was there a deficiency of acetylcholine synthesis by the nerve (presynaptic), excess of cholinesterase in the junction (synaptic), or a block of acetylcholine activity at the muscle endplate (post-synaptic)? This chapter explores the efforts to arrive at an answer to this question.

   Mary Walker and her pharmacologist, **Philip Hamill**, offered the hypothesis in 1935 that *"in myasthenia gravis there is a defective production at the nerve terminals of acetylcholine or some allied substance, and under the influence of the drug (Prostigmin) destruction of the substance is delayed."* In addition to this anti-cholinesterase action, physostigmine and "Prostigmin" were thought at the time to have an additional anti-curare action at the muscle endplate.[1] That these drugs had both an anti-cholinesterase and an anti-curare action was still the opinion in 1954 when a new drug, pyridostigmine bromide (Mestinon), was introduced into the United States by **Kermit Osserman**, **Paul Teng** and **L.I. Kaplan** for the treatment of myasthenia gravis.[2] So even the medicines used to treat myasthenia did not provide a specific answer as to why patients with myasthenia become weak.

Early indirect evidence for a postsynaptic defect, 1941-1956

Although Jolly had qualitatively demonstrated myasthenic muscle fatigue by tetanic faradic stimulation in 1895 (see pages 6 & 7), **A.M. Harvey** and **Richard Masland** at the University of Pennsylvania developed a quantitative method of supramaximal repetitive nerve stimulation in 1941 which demonstrated[3] that the response to muscles of myasthenic patients (see figure 3 on the right from their paper) was similar to that of partially curarized muscles, a resemblance first pointed out by Oppenheim in 1901. Curare was considered to compete with acetylcholine for the muscle endplate and thereby block acetylcholine stimulation of muscle. Similarities between myasthenia and curare, including the clinical picture, the electrical response and drug actions, induced Harvey and Masland to conclude that the defect in myasthenia gravis was in the muscle fiber or its motor endplate. In 1943 **A.E. Bennett** of the University of Nebraska showed that myasthenics were much more sensitive than others to curare.[4]

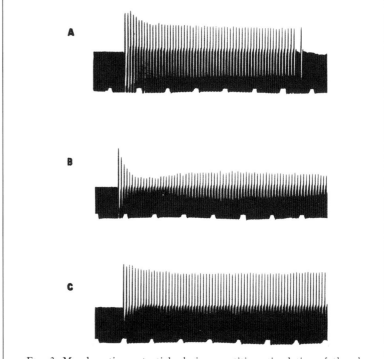

FIG. 3. Muscle action potentials during repetitive stimulation of the ulnar nerve, in a patient with myasthenia gravis. (A) Initial tetanus after rest. (B) Second tetanus ten seconds after the first. (C) Same as (B) thirty minutes after prostigmin. All nerve stimuli supramaximal. Time 0.2 sec. Initial potential 6.0 millivolts.

In contrast to their sensitivity to curare, some muscles of patients with myasthenia were shown by **H.C. Churchill-Davidson** and **A.T. Richardson** from St. Thomas's Hospital in London in 1953 to be several times more tolerant than normal muscles to a new "acetylcholine-like" drug, decamethonium iodide, that depolarized the muscle endplate like acetylcholine but was not destroyed by cholinesterase and therefore blocked neuromuscular transmission for many minutes.[5] Other myasthenic muscles had a different response to decamethonium, becoming rapidly paralyzed, but this paralysis could be reversed by anticholinesterases in myasthenic but not normal muscles. Churchill-Davidson called this a "dual response" which was interpreted as a myasthenic alteration of the response of the motor endplate to acetylcholine.

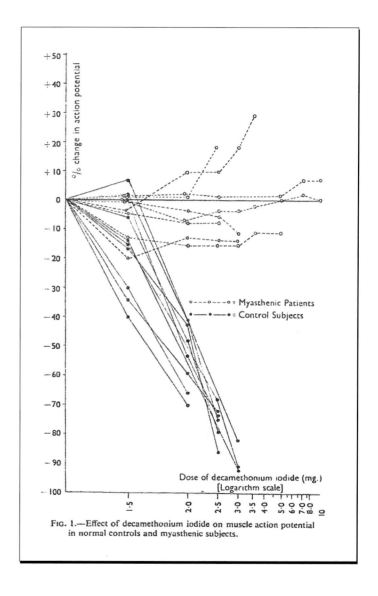

FIG. 1.—Effect of decamethonium iodide on muscle action potential in normal controls and myasthenic subjects.

A somewhat similar "dual response" was obtained from myasthenic muscles by intra-arterial injection of acetylcholine, reported[6] by **David Grob**, **Richard Johns** and **Harvey** at Johns Hopkins in 1956. Immediately after injection of acetylcholine a transient stimulation of muscles occurred, followed by brief failure of muscle activity. Recovery occurred within a minute but was soon followed by a second failure of neuromuscular transmission lasting thirty minutes or longer which was more marked than occurred in normal subjects and was reversible by acetylcholine or neostigmine in contrast to the additive depressant effect these agents produce in normal muscle (See fig. XIX below). This second failure of neuromuscular transmission could be mimicked by intra-arterial injection of high doses of choline, a breakdown product of acetylcholine, or of decamethonium, suggesting to these investigators that agents that depolarize normal muscle produce in myasthenic muscle an initial depolarization followed rapidly by a more marked and prolonged non-depolarizing (competitive) block. This was interpreted as evidence that the mechanism at fault in myasthenia was a decreased response of motor endplates to depolarization by acetylcholine or a product of acetylcholine.

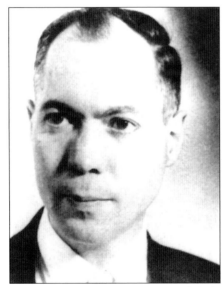

David Grob

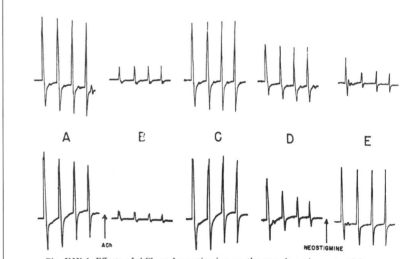

Fig. XIX.1. Effects of ACh and neostigmine on the muscle action potential response to nerve stimulation in a normal subject (*upper row*) and a patient with myasthenia gravis (*lower row*). A., control response to four supramaximal nerve stimuli at 40-msec. intervals; B., prompt depression 7 seconds after the intra-arterial injection of 5 mg. of ACh; C., recovery 15 seconds after injection; D., late depression one hour after injection; E., effect of 0.5 mg. of neostigmine (2).

Early Indirect Evidence for a Presynaptic Defect, 1957-1964

Other electrical and pharmacological responses of myasthenic muscles suggested to **John Desmedt** at the University of Brussels in Belgium that a presynaptic defect was present in myasthenia gravis. We have already seen in Chapter 2 (page 26) the abnormal nerve endings that Desmedt and Coërs described as occurring in myasthenia. Desmedt was impressed that myasthenic muscle not only fatigued rapidly during stimulation but that this fatigue also persisted after stimulation ceased, unlike curarized muscle. He argued in 1957 that this *"post-activation exhaustion"* might result from a depletion and deficient resynthesis of preformed acetyl-choline in nerve endings.[7] He added that it might also result from *"an enduring alteration of the chemoreceptor mechanism at the end-plate."* In 1958 Desmedt opted for the former possibility on the basis of the myasthenic-like features of neuromuscular transmission which occurred after the administration of a new chemical compound, the hemicholinium base HC3, which strongly inhibits synthesis of acetylcholine in nervous tissue by interfering with the supply of choline.[8]

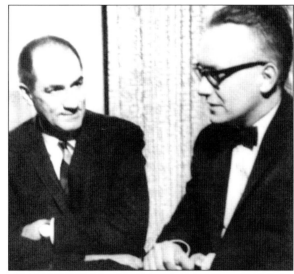

Edward Lambert and John Desmedt at the Third International Myasthenia Gravis Symposium, New York, 1965.

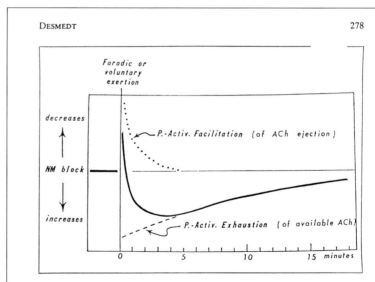

*Fig.*19. Diagram of proposed hypothesis of the dual nature of the myasthenic postactivation cycle with the changes in NM block after exercise (——) analyzed into facilitation (......) and exhaustion (– – – –) components [DESMEDT, 1961a].

S tructural study of the neuromuscular junction was greatly aided by the commercial availability of the electron microscope in the 1950's, as demonstrated below on the left by an electron-micrograph of the nerve terminal and muscle endplate of a snake. This photograph also contains on its right side a photomicrograph to scale of a salt-filled glass microelectrode, the technological advance that allowed fundamental understanding of the subcellular events which occur during neuromuscular transmission. These are demonstrated below on the right with a 1952 illustration from a benchmark paper in the *Journal of Physiology* by **Paul Fatt** and **Bernard Katz** of University College in London.[9]

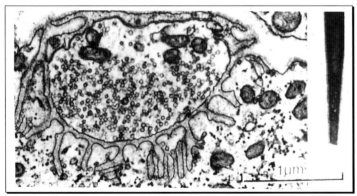

Electron micrograph: Nerve terminal and muscle endplate of a snake, with a glass micropipette pictured to scale on right.

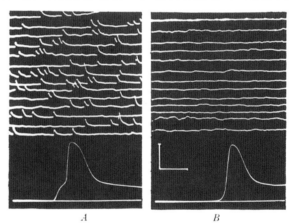

Fig. 1. Localization of spontaneous activity. M. ext. l. dig. IV. Intracellular recording. Part *A* was recorded at the end-plate, part *B* at a distance 2 mm away, in the same muscle fibre. The lower part, taken at high speed and low amplification, shows the response to a nerve stimulus (shock applied at beginning of sweep); the upper part, taken at low speed and high amplification, shows the spontaneous activity at the end-plate. Voltage and time scales: 50 mV and 2 msec for the lower part, and 3·6 mV and 47 msec for the upper part.

In 1964 **Dan Elmqvist**, **W.W. Hofmann**, **Jan Kugelberg** and **D.M.J. Quastel** at the University of Lund in Sweden used glass microelectrodes to record intracellularly from intercostal muscle biopsies obtained from humans, some of whom had myasthenia gravis.[10] They discovered that the mean amplitude of miniature endplate potentials measured near the endplate in myasthenic muscle was one-fifth that of non-myasthenic muscle (See fig. 5 below). This could be the result of any deficiency "upstream" from the muscle, presynaptic, synaptic, or postsynaptic. When bathed with acetylcholine-like drugs (carbachol) and decamethonium, however, the sensitivity of the myasthenic muscle endplates in these biopsies seemed to be similar to normal. From this Elmqvist and colleagues reasoned that the lesion in MG was presynaptic: *"In myasthenia there is a deficiency in the amount of acetylcholine in the transmitter quantum, probably brought about by a defect in the quantum formation mechanism or by the presence of a 'false transmitter.'"* Eventually these experiments would be repeated by others using much smaller amounts of these drugs applied by glass micropipettes right at the muscle endplate to obtain a different answer,[11] but for a decade the physiological data of Elmquist *et al* favored a presynaptic defect as responsible for the weakness in myasthenia gravis.

J. Physiol. (1964), 174, *pp.* 417–434
With 10 *text-figures*
Printed in Great Britain

417

AN ELECTROPHYSIOLOGICAL INVESTIGATION OF NEURO-
MUSCULAR TRANSMISSION IN MYASTHENIA GRAVIS

BY D. ELMQVIST, W. W. HOFMANN,* J. KUGELBERG
AND D. M. J. QUASTEL†

*From the Departments of Pharmacology and Thoracic Surgery.
University of Lund, Sweden*

(*Received* 22 *April* 1964)

Myasthenia gravis is a disease, described only in man, which is characterized by rapidly developing neuromuscular blockade during repetitive motor nerve activity. The mechanism underlying this block has remained obscure, despite a considerable amount of work on the subject (for reviews see Osserman, 1958; Foldes & McNall, 1962). By means of conventional electrophysiological techniques, with intracellular micro-electrodes to record from human intercostal muscle fibres *in vitro*, it has been possible to establish that the process of neuromuscular transmission in man is essentially similar to that in other mammalian species (Elmqvist, Johns & Thesleff, 1960). The same methods have been used in the present investigation to compare various aspects of the transmission process in specimens of myasthenic and normal intercostal muscle, obtained either at thoracotomy or by biopsy.

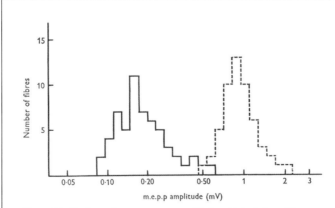

Fig. 5. Distributions of mean m.e.p.p. amplitudes obtained from fifty-seven myasthenic and fifty-four normal fibres in normal bathing mediums. All amplitudes corrected to a membrane potential of 85 mV. Full line myasthenic fibres, broken line normal fibres. Noise level was usually 50–100 μV.

SUMMARY

1. By the use of intracellular electrodes the neuromuscular transmission mechanism has been studied in isolated intercostal muscle obtained from patients with myasthenia gravis.

2. On repetitive nerve stimulation at frequencies above 2/sec, only the first few stimuli elicited muscle contractions in most fibres and then subthreshold end-plate potentials (e.p.p.s) could be recorded.

3. Miniature end-plate potentials (m.e.p.p.s) had a mean amplitude of 0·2 mV, one fifth of the normal. The calculated size of the quantal components of e.p.p.s corresponded closely to the m.e.p.p. amplitude.

4. The average resting frequency of m.e.p.p.s was 0·2/sec, the same as in normal human intercostal muscle, and the frequency was increased by nerve stimulation and by potassium. The quantum content of e.p.p.s at various frequencies of nerve stimulation was similar to that at normal junctions.

5. Post-synaptic chemosensitivity, as tested by bath-application of carbachol and decamethonium, was normal. The input resistance of the fibres in myasthenic muscle was about 0·5 MΩ, the same as in normal muscle. Resting membrane potential of myasthenic fibres was also normal.

6. It is tentatively concluded that in myasthenia gravis there is a deficiency in the amount of acetylcholine in the quanta of transmitter released from the motor nerve terminals.

The Ultrastructure of the Human Neuromuscular Junction

This illustration from a 1972 paper from the Mayo Clinic in Rochester, Minnesota, shows the variability in the appearance under the electron microscope of normal human neuromuscular junctions, compared to that from a patient with myasthenia gravis (next page).

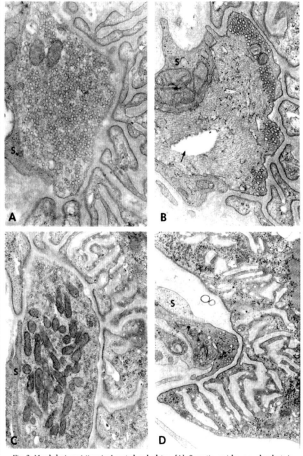

Normal neuromuscular junctions

Fig. 3. Morphologic variations in 4 control end plates. [A] Synaptic vesicles are abundant in nerve terminal. × 26,800. [B] Synaptic vesicles are sparse, clear space in axon (arrow) is preparatory artifact. × 30,600. [C] Nerve terminal is large and contains many mitochondria. × 20,300. [D] Nerve terminal is small. Small myelin figure and few dark glycogen granules appear in nerve terminal, and a portion of terminal is completely surrounded by Schwann cells. Secondary synaptic clefts are deeper and postsynaptic membrane is more complex than in [C]. × 21,400. S = Schwann cell.

At the level of the electron microscope, definite abnormalities of the neuromuscular junction in myasthenia gravis could finally be seen. In a careful quantitative study of neuromuscular junction ultrastructure in intercostal muscles from normal controls and patients with myasthenia gravis, reported in 1972 by **Tetsuji Santa**, **Andrew Engel**, and **Edward Lambert** of the Mayo Clinic,[12] the mean presynaptic vesicle diameter and vesicle count per unit nerve terminal area of MG endplates were not significantly different from normal, but both the mean presynaptic nerve terminal area and the postsynaptic membrane folds and clefts were decreased and the synaptic cleft was widened in myasthenia gravis (Tables 1 & 2). Initially, therefore, electron microscopy failed to resolve whether the location of the lesion in myasthenia gravis was presynaptic, synaptic or postsynaptic. The answer, however, was soon to follow.

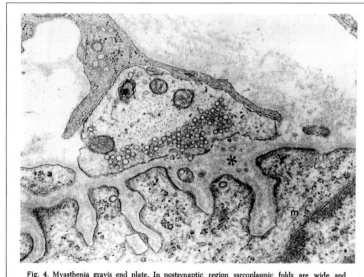

Fig. 4. Myasthenia gravis end plate. In postsynaptic region sarcoplasmic folds are wide and secondary synaptic clefts sparse. Loosely arranged junctional sarcoplasm contains microtubules and ribosomes. Asterisk indicates widening of primary synaptic cleft. m = microtubule. × 39,600.

Neuromuscular junction of a patient with myasthenia gravis, as viewed by the electron microscope. The asterisk marks the widened synaptic cleft.

TABLE 1

HISTOMETRIC ANALYSIS OF NERVE TERMINALS*

	Area (sq. μ)	Mitochondrial area (%)	Vesicles per sq. μ	Vesicle diameter (Ångströms)
Control	3.92 ± 0.4 (No. = 63)	18.1 ± 1.5 (No. = 51)	50.3 ± 3.6 (No. = 59)	560.8 ± 2.8 (No. = 1,133)
Myasthenia gravis	2.28 ± 0.2† (No. = 112)	16.6 ± 1.3 (No. = 100)	46.3 ± 2.8 (No. = 104)	568.2 ± 4.9 (No. = 1,420)

No. indicates the number of nerve terminals analyzed except in the last column where it refers to the number of vesicle diameters. More than one nerve terminal can be found in an end plate.
* Values indicate mean ± SE.
† Significant difference from control value (p < 0.05)

TABLE 2

HISTOMETRIC ANALYSIS OF POSTSYNAPTIC REGION*

	Area per nerve terminal (sq. μ)	Membrane profile concentration (μ/sq. μ)	PostSML / PreSML
Control	10.58 ± 0.79 (No. = 54)	5.83 ± 0.25 (No. = 47)	10.10 ± 0.75 (No. = 39)
Myasthenia gravis	6.55 ± 0.36† (No. = 108)	3.95 ± 0.21† (No. = 87)	8.04 ± 0.72 (No. = 85)

No. indicates the number of areas analyzed. Postsynaptic region here refers to area of folds and clefts per nerve terminal. More than one such region can be found in an end plate.
* Values indicate mean ± SE.
† Significant difference from control value (p < 0.05)

Two "Gifts of Nature"

The snake venoms of cobras and kraits and the electric organs of the electric eel and torpedo fish were essential for unraveling the mystery of why patients with myasthenia gravis are weak. Worldwide scientific investigations of these two "gifts of nature," to use **David Richman's** felicitous phrase,[13] initially contributed basic understanding of normal neuromuscular transmission and eventually helped elucidate the basic neuromuscular defect underlying myasthenia.

A particular neurotoxin called "alpha-bungarotoxin" was isolated from the venom of the many-ringed Formosan krait, *Bungarus multicinctus*, by **Chuan-Chiung Chang** and **Chen-Yuan Lee** of National Taiwan University[14] in 1963. Unlike curare, which binds only temporarily at the neuromuscular junction, alpha-bungarotoxin bound not only specifically but nearly irreversibly to motor endplates,[15] as demonstrated by **Lee, L.F. Tseng** and **T.H. Chiu** in 1967. This meant that it could be "labeled" with radioactivity to identify motor endplates variously processed for research purposes.

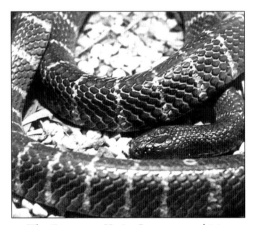

The Formosan Krait, *Bungarus multicinctus*

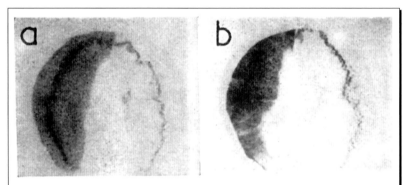

Fig. 1. Effect of phrenicotomy on fixation by α-bungarotoxin labelled with iodine-131 after 14 days (*a*) and 60 days (*b*). Right side: innervated hemidiaphragm; left side: phrenicotomized hemidiaphragm. Each rat was injected subcutaneously with 0·3 µg/g of α-bungarotoxin and died at 75 min (*a*) and 110 min (*b*) respectively after the injection.

A figure from the 1967 paper by Lee, Tseng & Chiu,[15] showing diaphragm muscles of two rats. On the right side of each diaphragm the normal condition is shown, with alpha-bungarotoxin staining only a line of neuromuscular junctions. The phrenic nerve to the left side of each diaphragm has been cut, after which alpha-bungarotoxin binding occurs throughout the muscle.

Because the electric organs of fish have evolved from neuromuscular junctions, they contain large quantities of proteins also found in motor endplates, an attribute that makes them suitable for biochemical analyses. Radioactive alpha-bungarotoxin was used in 1970 by **Lee** with **Jean-Pierre Changeux** and **Michiki Kasai** from the Institut Pasteur in Paris to characterize the cholinergic (acetylcholine) receptor macromolecule in the electric organs of the electric eel, *Electrophorus electricus*,[16] and also by **R. Miledi**, **P. Molinoff** and **L.T. Potter** at University College London in 1971 to isolate and purify cholinergic receptors from *Torpedo marmorata*.[17]

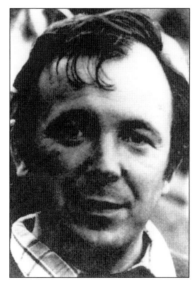

Jean-Pierre Changeux at Cold
Spring Harbor, 1975

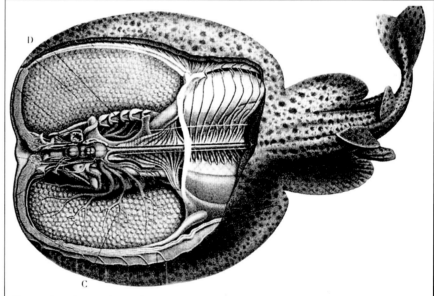

Fig. 3 - *Dorsal view of Torpedo Galvani.*

D,C - Electric Organs: the dorsal part has been ablated on the left electric organ (c). in order to show the nerves which innervate the electric organ (From Paolo Savi. *Etudes anatomiques sur le système nerveux et sur l'organe électrique de la torpille*, published at the end of Matteucci's *Traité des phénomènes électro-physiologiques des animaux*, Paris. Fortin et Masson. 1844, pl. I, fig. 1.

I n Baltimore, Maryland, in 1972 **Douglas Fambrough** of the Carnegie Institution and **Criss Hartzell** of the Johns Hopkins University compared the specific locations of radioactive alpha-bungarotoxin and the endplate marker acetylcholinesterase (AChE) in single muscle fibers from rats and revealed that virtually all of the acetylcholine receptors, labeled with alpha-bungarotoxin, were localized in the postsynaptic endplate.[18]

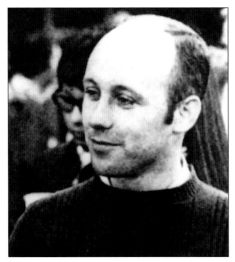

Douglas Fambrough at Cold Spring
Harbor, 1975

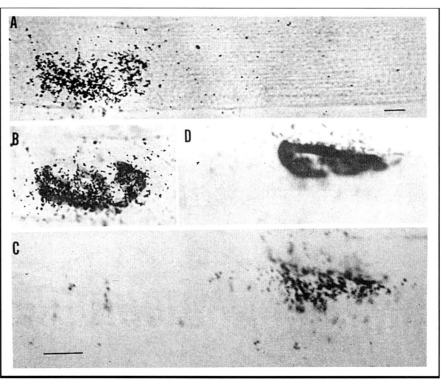

Autoradiographs of the end plate regions of isolated muscle fibers that had been incubated with [^{125}I]a-BGT. One end plate is shown before (A) and after (B) the preparation was stained for AChE; a second end plate is also seen oriented toward one side of the fiber, before (C) and after (D) staining for AChE. Magnification bars in (A) and (C) represent 10 µm.

(Reprinted with permission from Fambrough and Hartzell, *Science* 176: 189-190, copyright 1972 by American Association for the Advancement of Science.)

These tools were applied almost immediately to the elucidation of the pathogenesis of myasthenia gravis. In 1973 Fambrough with **Daniel Drachman** and **S. Satyamurti** of Johns Hopkins University used the same technique on human muscle fibers and demonstrated that the number of junctional acetylcholine receptors in myasthenic muscles was reduced to 11-30% of that in normal control muscles.[19] They speculated that this reduction in receptors might account for the defect in neuromuscular transmission in myasthenia gravis.

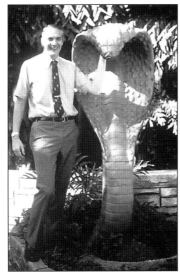

Daniel Drachman at Miami Serpentarium

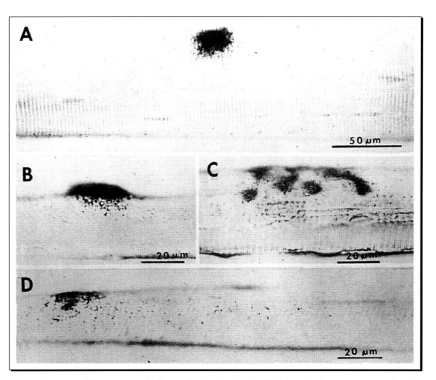

Autoradiograms of human muscle fibers after incubation in ^{125}I-labeled *a*-bungarotoxin and staining for acetylcholinesterase to reveal neuromuscular junctions. (A & B) Normal fibers from two patients (H.H. & N.A.). There is a dense accumulation of silver grains over a limited junctional area and a paucity of grains outside this region. (C) Myasthenic fiber (patient A.N.). The number of grains is markedly reduced, but grains are mostly localized over cholinesterase-stained area. (D) Myasthenic fibers (patient F.S.) showing decreased grain density at neuromuscular junction and a relatively high grain density over the adjacent extrajunctional region.

(Reprinted with permission from Fambrough et al, *Science* 182: 193-195, copyright 1973 by American Association for the Advancement of Science.)

Antibodies to the Acetylcholine Receptor

Meanwhile, at the Salk Institute in La Jolla, two basic scientists were interested in studying the structure of the acetylcholine receptor protein highly purified from *Electrophorus electricus.* As part of their investigation, **Jim Patrick** and **Jon Lindstrom** injected purified eel receptor into rabbits in order to produce antibodies to the eel receptor. Several of these rabbits died; others developed a flaccid paralysis and respiratory distress which could be temporarily reversed by neostigmine bromide ("Prostigmin").[20] Their muscles showed a decremental response to repetitive nerve stimulation which could also be reversed by neostigmine, similar to myasthenia gravis.

Experimental immunization with acetylcholine receptor seemed to have produced a model disease resembling myasthenia gravis which is called "experimental autoimmune myasthenia gravis" (EAMG) and which has been useful in elucidating the pathogenesis of MG. Assuming that the eel receptor had caused the rabbits to produce not only an immune response to eel receptor but also an autoimmune response to their own rabbit acetylcholine receptors, these authors speculated that myasthenia gravis might be a consequence of an autoimmune response to human acetylcholine receptors.

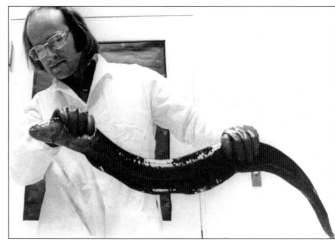

Jon Lindstrom with *Electrophorus electricus* (note rubber gloves).

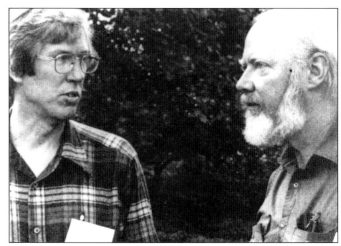

Jim Patrick and M.A. Raftery at Cold Spring Harbor, 1983.

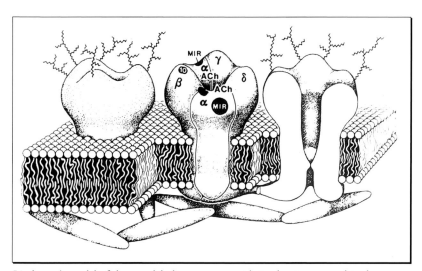

Lindstrom's model of the acetylcholine receptor, with 5 subunits arranged in the membrane around an ion pore and 2 sites for acetylcholine binding.

These rabbits, pictured in Patrick & Lindstrom's 1973 article in *Science*, had antibodies not only to *Electrophorus* electric organ receptor but also to rabbit acetylcholine receptor. Their weakness and decremental responses could be alleviated by edrophonium or neostigmine, as suggested by Dr. Vanda Lennon.

(Reprinted with permission from Patrick and Lindstrom, *Science* 180: 871-872, copyright 1973 by American Association for the Advancement of Science.)

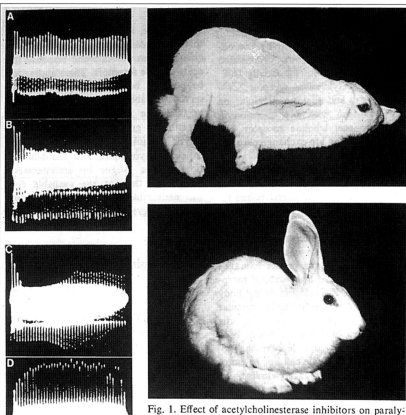

Fig. 1. Effect of acetylcholinesterase inhibitors on paralysis and electromyograms. (Right) The upper photograph shows a rabbit 5 days after the third injection of acetylcholine receptor. The bottom photograph is of the same animal 1 minute after receiving 0.3 mg of edrophonium intravenously. (Left) Electromyograms, before and after neostigmine injection, were taken on a control rabbit and on the rabbit seen on the right. Records were taken from a rear leg at a stimulus frequency of 40 per second. (A) Control before neostigmine; (B) experimental animal before neostigmine; (C) control after neostigmine; (D) experimental animal after neostigmine.

Several investigators therefore began to look for acetylcholine receptor antibodies in the sera of humans with myasthenia gravis. In 1974 **Richard Almon**, **Clifford Andrew** and **Stanley Appel** at Duke University in North Carolina reported that serum globulin from at least one-third of patients with myasthenia gravis significantly inhibited the binding of alpha-bungarotoxin to acetylcholine receptors extracted from denervated rat muscles.[21] This was confirmed by immunohistochemistry on human muscle by **Adam Bender**, **Steven Ringel**, **W. King Engel**, **Mathew Daniels** and **Zvi Vogel** from the National Institutes of Health in Bethesda, Maryland, in 1975,[22] 44% of myasthenic sera blocking the binding of immunoperoxidase-labelled alpha-bungarotoxin to muscle endplates. **Appel**, **Almon** and **Nelson Levy** at Duke, using a radioimmunoprecipitation assay, reported in 1975 the presence of antibodies to *rat* acetylcholine receptor in 30% of patients with myasthenia gravis.[23] A similar assay using *human* acetylcholine receptor demonstrated that 87% of sera from patients with myasthenia gravis had elevated amounts of antibodies specific for human acetylcholine receptors, compared to no elevation in non-myasthenic sera.[24] This was reported in 1976 by **Lindstrom** with **Vanda Lennon** at the Salk Institute, **Marjorie Seybold** from the University of California at San Diego, **Senga Whitingham** from Melbourne, Australia, and **Drake Duane** from the Mayo Clinic.

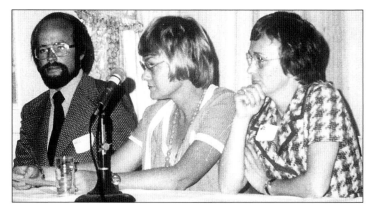

Drs. Jon Lindstrom, Vanda Lennon, and Marjorie Seybold.

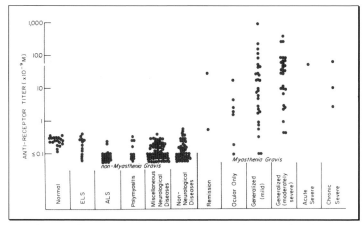

Distribution of antireceptor antibody titers in subjects with and without myasthenia gravis. ELS = Eaton-Lambert syndrome, ALS = amyotrophic lateral sclerosis.

Myasthenia as an Antibody-mediated Autoimmune Disease

These previous studies established that measureable antibodies to acetylcholine receptor were present in the blood of many but not all patients with myasthenia gravis and that these antibodies interacted with the target antigen, the muscle acetylcholine receptor. Another criterion for an antibody-mediated autoimmune disease – that reduction in antibodies ameliorates the disease – was first shown in London, England, in 1976 by **A.J. Pinching** and **D.K. Peters** from Hammersmith Hospital together with **John Newsom-Davis** from the National Hospital for Nervous Diseases.[25] They gave three patients with myasthenia gravis daily plasma exchanges, removing the serum containing all the immunoglobulin antibodies and replacing it with albumin and saline solution. These patients improved clinically. The increases in the vital capacity of the lungs and the length of time during which arms could be outstretched were documented.

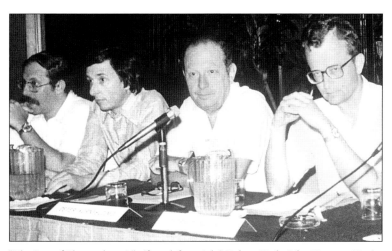

"The Joys of Plasmapheresis": (from left to right) Robert Lisak, John Newsom-Davis, Peter Kornfeld, and Peter Dau at a MG Plasmapheresis conference, June, 1978.

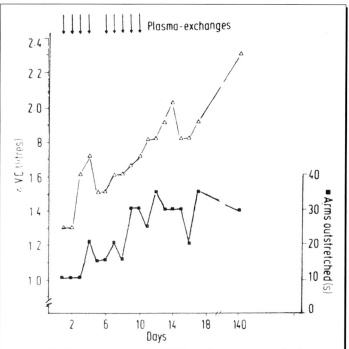

Fig. 1 Daily measurements of V.C. and arm-outstretched time in case 1.
Immunosuppression was started on day 16. Arrows mark the plasma-exchanges, which averaged 1 litre in the first week and 2 litres in the second.

One final criterion for antibody-mediated autoimmune disease – that passive transfer of antibodies could reproduce the disease features – was provided by **Klaus Toyka**, **Dan Drachman**, **Ing Kao**, and others, who showed at Johns Hopkins University in 1977 that passive transfer of immunoglobulin antibodies from myasthenic patients to mice could reproduce the disease features in these mice.[26] However, these latter two studies did not identify the specific antibodies that might be causing weakness. Very recent findings suggest that those patients without serum antibodies to acetylcholine receptors may instead have antibodies to other proteins at the neuromuscular junction such as muscle-specific kinase (MuSK).[27]

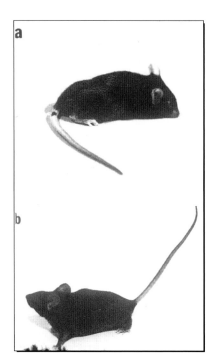

Clinical weakness in a recipient mouse:
The mouse in (a) received the crude immunoglobulin fraction from Case 8 for eight days. A control mouse (b) received pooled normal immunoglobulin for eight days.

(Reprinted with permission from Toyka et al, *New England J Med* 296: 125-131, copyright 1977, Massachusetts Medical Society. All rights reserved.)

THE 1970'S WAS A REMARKABLE DECADE in the history of myasthenia gravis, every year bringing an important advance. Although significant contributions continued to pour forth from many of the above investigators in subsequent years, by 1977 the autoimmune pathogenesis of myasthenia gravis, at least at the neuromuscular junction, had been clearly established. This information also helped the elucidation of less well understood related conditions, described in the next chapter.

References for Chapter 5: Presnaptic, Synaptic, or Postsynaptic? (1935-1977)

1. Hamill P, Walker MB: The action of "Prostigmin" (Roche) in neuro-muscular disorders. *J Physiology* 82:36P-37P, 1935.

2. Osserman KE, Teng P, Kaplan LI: Studies in myasthenia gravis. Preliminary report on therapy with Mestinon bromide. *J of the American Medical Association* 155:961-965, 1954.

3. Harvey AM, Masland RL: The electromyogram in myasthenia gravis. *Bulletin of Johns Hopkins Hospital* 69:1-13, 1941.

4. Bennett AE, Cash PB: Myasthenia gravis – curare sensitivity, a new diagnostic test and approach to causation. *Archives of Neurology & Psychiatry* 49:537-547, 1943.

5. Churchill-Davidson HC, Richardson AT: The action of decamethonium iodide (C.10) in myasthenia gravis. *J Neurology, Neurosurgery, & Psychiatry* 15:129-133, 1952.

6. Grob D, Johns RJ, Harvey AM: Studies in neuromuscular function IV. Stimulating and depressant effects of acetylcholine and choline in patients with myasthenia gravis, and their relationship to the defect in neuromuscular transmission. *Bulletin of Johns Hopkins Hospital* 99:153-181, 1956.

7. Desmedt JE: Nature of the defect of neuromuscular transmission in myasthenic patients: "Post-tetanic exhaustion." *Nature* (London) 179:156-157, 1957.

8. Desmedt JE: Myasthenic-like features of neuromuscular transmission after administration of an inhibitor of acetylcholine synthesis. *Nature* (London) 182:1673-1674, 1958.

9. Fatt P, Katz B: Spontaneous subthreshold activity at motor nerve endings. *J Physiology* (London) Volume #117:109-128, 1952.

10. Elmqvist D, Hofmann WW, Kugelberg J, Quastel DMJ: An electrophysiological investigation of neuromuscular transmission in myasthenia gravis. *J Physiology* (London) 174:417-434, 1964.

11. Albuquerque EX, Rash JE, Mayer RF, Satterfield JR: An electrophysiological and morphological study of the neuromuscular junction in patients with myasthenia gravis. *Experimental Neurology* 51:536-563, 1976.

12. Santa T, Engel AG, Lambert EH: Histometric study of neuromuscular junction ultrastructure I. Myasthenia gravis. *Neurology* 22:71-82, 1972.

13. Richman DP, Agius MA: Acquired myasthenia gravis, immunopathology. *Neurology Clinics of North America* 12:273-284, 1994.

14. Chang CC, Lee CY: Isolation of neurotoxins from the venom of Bungarus multicinctus and their modes of neuromuscular blocking action. *Archives of International Pharmacodynamics* 144:241-257, 1963.

continued...

...*continued*

15. Lee CY, Tseng LF, Chiu TH: Influence of denervation on localization of neurotoxins from clapid venoms in rat diaphragm. *Nature* (London) 215:1177-1178, 1967.

16. Changeux JP, Kasai M, Lee CY: Use of a snake venom toxin to characterize the cholinergic receptor protein. *Proceedings of the National Academy of Sciences* 67:1241-1247, 1970.

17. Miledi R, Molinoff P, Potter LT: Isolation of the cholinergic receptor protein of Torpedo electric tissue. *Nature* (London) 229:554-557, 1971.

18. Fambrough DM, Hartzell HC: Acetylcholine receptors: Number and distribution at neuromuscular junctions in rat diaphragm. *Science* 176:189-190, 1972.

19. Fambrough DM, Drachman DB, Satyamurti S: Neuromuscular junction in myasthenia gravis: Decreased acetylcholine receptors. *Science* 182:193-195, 1973.

20. Patrick J, Lindstrom J: Autoimmune response to acetylcholine receptor. *Science* 180:871-872, 1973.

21. Almon RR, Andrew CG, Appel SH: A serum globulin in myasthenia gravis: Inhibition of alpha-bungarotoxin binding to acetylcholine receptors. *Science* 186:55-57, 1974.

22. Bender AN, Ringel SP, Engel WK, Daniels MP, Vogel Z: Myasthenia gravis: A serum factor blocking acetylcholine receptors of the human neuromuscular junction. *Lancet* 1:607-609, 1975.

23. Appel SH, Almon RR, Levy N: Acetylcholine receptor antibodies in myasthenia gravis. *New England J of Medicine* 293:760-761, 1975.

24. Lindstrom JM, Seybold ME, Lennon VA, Whittingham S, Duane DD: Antibody to acetylcholine receptor in myasthenia gravis. *Neurology* 26:1054-1059, 1976.

25. Pinching AJ, Peters DK, Newsom-Davis J: Remission of myasthenia gravis following plasma exchange. *Lancet* 2:1373-1376, 1976.

26. Toyka KV, Drachman DB, Griffith DE, Winkelstein JA, Fischbeck KH, Kao I: Study of humoral immune mechanisms by passive transfer to mice. *N England J of Medicine* 296:125-130, 1977.

27. Hoch W, McConville J, Helms S, Newsom-Davis J, Melms A, Vincent A: Auto-antibodies to the receptor tyrosine kinase MuSK in patients with myasthenia gravis without acetylcholine receptor antibodies. *Nature Medicine* 7:365-368, 2001.

6 Related Disorders (1937-1990)

Introduction

Other conditions resembling myasthenia gravis exist which eventually were shown *not* to be associated with measurable antibodies to muscle acetylcholine receptor. This chapter will briefly describe the histories of these entities, which are still evolving.

One of these, distinguished from classical myasthenia gravis years before the acetylcholine receptor antibody was discovered, became known as the **Lambert-Eaton Myasthenic Syndrome**. It has recently turned out to be an autoimmune disease of the presynaptic terminal, mirroring myasthenia gravis, an autoimmune disease of the postsynaptic membrane.

The other group of conditions is inherited, not autoimmune. It includes a variety of myasthenias that manifest themselves shortly after birth and have come to be known as **Congenital Myasthenic Syndromes**.

Lambert-Eaton Myasthenic Syndrome, 1951-1989

THE LANCET]   [DEC. 19, 1953 1291

BRONCHIAL NEOPLASM WITH MYASTHENIA
PROLONGED APNŒA AFTER ADMINISTRATION OF SUCCINYLCHOLINE

H. J. ANDERSON
M.B. Camb., F.R.C.P.
CONSULTANT PHYSICIAN, DEPARTMENT OF THORACIC MEDICINE

H. C. CHURCHILL-DAVIDSON
M.A., M.D. Camb., D.A.
WILL EDMONDS RESEARCH FELLOW OF THE ROYAL COLLEGE
OF PHYSICIANS, DEPARTMENT OF ANÆSTHETICS

A. T. RICHARDSON
M.B. Lond., M.R.C.P., D.Phys.Med.
SENIOR REGISTRAR, DEPARTMENT OF PHYSICAL MEDICINE

ST. THOMAS'S HOSPITAL, LONDON

In a 1953 paper first-authored by **H.J. Anderson**[1] the physicians from St. Thomas's Hospital whom we encountered in the previous chapter, **H.C. Churchill-Davidson** and **A.T. Richardson**, described a patient with a bronchial neoplasm seen at that hospital in 1951 in whom severe muscle weakness disappeared almost immediately after removal of the tumor, suggesting *"that such neoplasms might give rise to an unusual form of peripheral neuropathy, possibly similar to myasthenia gravis."* They investigated another case in 1953, a 47-year-old man with leg weakness, fatigue and decreased deep tendon reflexes but without ptosis or dysarthria, whose response to decamethonium, d-tubocurarine, succinylcholine and neostigmine was *"similar to that seen in myasthenia gravis."*

The following year, in a pathological review of 19 patients with "Carcinomatous neuropathy and myopathy," **R.A. Henson**, **Dorothy Russell**, and **Marcia Wilkinson** from The London Hospital reported five patients with carcinoma of the bronchus who exhibited neostigmine-responsive fatigue like that of myasthenia, but were different in having sensory complaints, decreased or absent deep tendon reflexes and early muscle wasting.[2] The adjacent article in the same issue of *Brain*, by **K.W.G. Heathfield** and **J.R.B. Williams** from St. Bartholomew's Hospital in London, described five cases of "Peripheral neuropathy and myopathy associated with bronchogenic carcinoma," among which was a 54-year-old man who, eighteen months *after* he developed decreased tendon reflexes and neostigmine-responsive hip and thigh weakness, was discovered to have a carcinoma of the lung.[3] Other papers at about the same time described similar patients.

Brain
A Journal of Neurology

Vol. 77.   Part I.   1954   Price 12s. 6d. net.
                                                       Subscription 50s. net.

82   CARCINOMATOUS NEUROPATHY AND MYOPATHY
         A CLINICAL AND PATHOLOGICAL STUDY[1]
                            BY
         R. A. HENSON, DOROTHY S. RUSSELL AND MARCIA WILKINSON
         (From the Wards and Bernhard Baron Institute of Pathology, The London Hospital)

122   PERIPHERAL NEUROPATHY AND MYOPATHY ASSOCIATED
         WITH BRONCHOGENIC CARCINOMA
                            BY
         K. W. G. HEATHFIELD AND J. R. B. WILLIAMS
         (From the Departments of Neurology and Pathology, St. Bartholomew's Hospital, London)

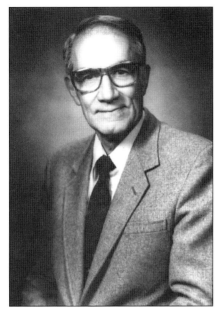

Edward H. Lambert

AMERICAN PHYSIOLOGICAL SOCIETY

PROCEEDINGS

FALL MEETING, SEPTEMBER 4-7, 1956

612

Defect of neuromuscular conduction associated with malignant neoplasms. EDWARD H. LAMBERT, LEE M. EATON* AND E. D. ROOKE.* Mayo Fndn., Rochester, Minn.

An unusual defect of neuromuscular conduction has been observed in 3 patients with positive evidence and 3 patients with suggestive evidence of malignant tumor in the chest. These patients had weakness of proximal muscles of the extremities, decreased or absent tendon reflexes and an increased fatigability which was suggestive of myasthenia gravis. Neostigmine caused only slight or equivocal improvement in strength, although the patients were very sensitive to *d*-tubocurarine. Electromyographic studies revealed that a single maximal shock to the ulnar nerve produced an action potential and twitch of muscles of the hand which were greatly reduced in amplitude (2-30% of normal), although the strength of these muscles on voluntary contraction was essentially normal. A transient further decline in response, like that seen in myasthenia gravis, occurred with the onset of repetitive stimulation at rates of 1-10/sec., but a marked facilitation of the response (up to 10 times the initial amplitude) occurred during continued repetitive stimulation at higher rates. A similar facilitation occurred during voluntary contraction. After a short rest the initial contraction was very weak, but increased to nearly normal strength in 15-45 sec. For several seconds after voluntary contractions, the response to electric stimulation of the nerve was increased up to 20 times the response prior to exercise. In some features of these and other studies the defect in neuromuscular response resembled that of myasthenia gravis, however the depression of the initial response and the phenomenon of facilitation were more marked than is usually observed in the latter disorder.

613

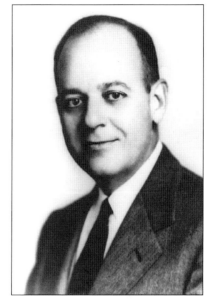

Lee M. Eaton

However, it was **Edward Lambert**, **Lee Eaton**, and **E. Douglas Rooke** of the Mayo Clinic in Rochester, Minnesota, who provided the definitive delineation of this myasthenic syndrome from other carcinomatous neuropathies and from myasthenia gravis. They reported "an unusual defect in neuromuscular conduction," observed in six patients with evidence for a malignant chest tumor,[4] at the Fall Meeting of the American Physiological Society in September, 1956. Rooke relates that whereas he examined limb muscle strength of these patients with a repetitive pumping motion and concluded that they became stronger, Eaton immediately overcame the patients' muscle resistance by manual force and thought that they were weak. They turned to the electrophysiologist Lambert for an explanation, and he demonstrated the characteristic electrophysiological findings of a decreased compound muscle action potential to a single stimulus (what Eaton initially examined clinically), and pronounced facilitation of the response to stimulation rates greater than 10 Hz (similar to Rooke's manner of repetitive examination).

In 1957, this new condition was referred to briefly at the end of a general review of electromyography in the *Journal of the American Medical Association* in which Eaton was the first author.[5] Sadly, Eaton died abruptly of a myocardial infarction on November 18, 1958, at the age of 53 years. He had chaired the Section of Neurology at the Mayo Clinic since 1955.

ELECTROMYOGRAPHY AND ELECTRIC STIMULATION
OF NERVES IN DISEASES OF MOTOR UNIT

OBSERVATIONS ON MYASTHENIC SYNDROME ASSOCIATED WITH MALIGNANT TUMORS

Lee M. Eaton, M.D.
and
Edward H. Lambert, M.D., Rochester, Minn.

1957

As a final example of the usefulness of electromyography in clinical research, we present descriptions of six patients who have a disorder resembling myasthenia gravis, which may represent a specific clinical-electromyographic syndrome. This has been of great interest to us, since in three of the six patients the diagnosis of malignant tumor has been established and in two others roentgenographic evidence suggesting intrathoracic malignant disease has been found. Investigations already under way should, in time, elucidate the significance of this neuromuscular disorder. Perhaps it may not be premature to discuss briefly the nature of this disorder as it has been observed thus far.

MYASTHENIC SYNDROME OCCASIONALLY
ASSOCIATED WITH BRONCHIAL
NEOPLASM: NEUROPHYSIOLOGIC
STUDIES °

1959

EDWARD H. LAMBERT, E. DOUGLAS ROOKE,
LEE M. EATON ** AND CORRIN H. HODGSON

In subsequent paragraphs the condition of myasthenia sometimes associated with bronchial neoplasm will be referred to as the "myasthenic syndrome S. C. Ca." (meaning "myasthenic syndrome sometimes associated with small cell bronchogenic carcinoma") to distinguish it from classic myasthenia gravis.

GENERAL CHARACTERISTICS OF THE
MYASTHENIC SYNDROME SOMETIMES ASSOCIATED WITH
SMALL CELL BRONCHOGENIC CARCINOMA

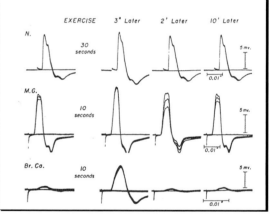

The first full description of the new syndrome called it "Myasthenic Syndrome S.C.Ca," meaning "myasthenic syndrome sometimes associated with small cell bronchogenic carcinoma!" This was presented at the *Second International MG Symposium* in Los Angeles in 1959, and published in the Proceedings of that meeting in 1961.[6] The suggested name was so awkward that it was soon replaced by "**Eaton-Lambert Syndrome**" and eventually by **Lambert-Eaton Myasthenic Syndrome**, or **LEMS** (See graph at right).

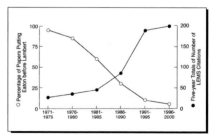

In 1968 further understanding of the Lambert-Eaton Myasthenic Syndrome was provided by an intracellular microelectrode study of muscle biopsies from patients with this syndrome. **Dan Elmqvist** from Sweden, while working with **Edward Lambert** at the Mayo Clinic, demonstrated that action potentials arriving at motor nerve terminals in LEMS biopsies produced an insufficient release of acetylcholine quanta,[7] but that this could be increased by repetitive stimulation during which more calcium entered the nerve terminal. Acetylcholine release could also be increased by increasing the extracellular calcium concentration. Both these procedures suggested that the defect in acetylcholine release in LEMS was caused by reduced calcium entry into motor nerve terminals. In the 1970's several laboratories demonstrated that the normal release of acetylcholine at active zones on the presynaptic membrane of the neuromuscular junction was dependent upon calcium.

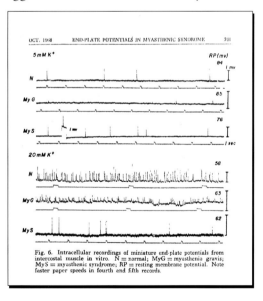

Fig. 6. Intracellular recordings of miniature end-plate potentials from intercostal muscle in vitro. N = normal; MyG = myasthenia gravis; MyS = myasthenic syndrome; RP = resting membrane potential. Note faster paper speeds in fourth and fifth records.

Ludwig Gutmann and his associates in 1972 were the first to draw attention to the association of LEMS with autoimmune disorders such as hypothyroidism and pernicious anemia.[9] Shortly thereafter, the first LEMS patient to benefit from plasmapheresis was reported by **Eric Denys** and **Peter Dau** from San Francisco, with **Jon Lindstrom**, at a 1978 symposium on plasmapheresis.[10]

By August 1981, **Bethan Lang**, **John Newsom-Davis**, **Dennis Wray**, and **Angela Vincent** from the Royal Free Hospital in London, with **Nicholas Murray** from London's National Hospital for Nervous Diseases, were able to hypothesize that LEMS might be an autoimmune disease of the pre-synaptic terminal on the basis of clinical improvement of three LEMS patients by plasma exchange or immunosuppressive treatment, with additional experimental evidence of electrophysiologic changes in mice injected with immunoglobulin from these patients.[11]

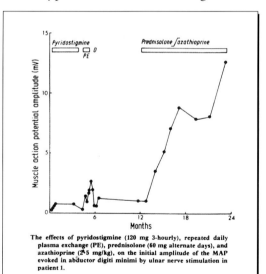

The effects of pyridostigmine (120 mg 3-hourly), repeated daily plasma exchange (PE), prednisolone (60 mg alternate days), and azathioprine (2.5 mg/kg), on the initial amplitude of the MAP evoked in abductor digiti minimi by ulnar nerve stimulation in patient 1.

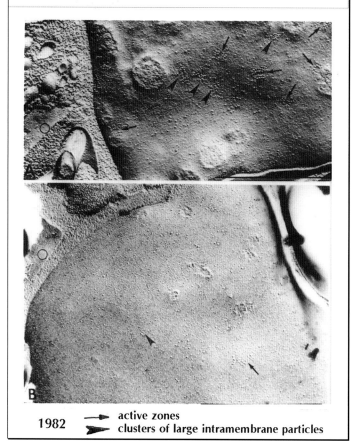

MUSCLE & NERVE 5:686–697 1982

PAUCITY AND DISORGANIZATION OF PRESYNAPTIC MEMBRANE ACTIVE ZONES IN THE LAMBERT-EATON MYASTHENIC SYNDROME

HIDETOSHI FUKUNAGA, MD, ANDREW G. ENGEL, MD, MITSUHIRO OSAME, MD, and EDWARD H. LAMBERT, MD

1982 → active zones
➤ clusters of large intramembrane particles

These hypotheses were strengthened in 1982 when the paucity and disorganization of the active zones on LEMS presynaptic membranes were visualized by **Hidetoshi Fukunaga**, **Andrew Engel**, **Mitsuhiro Osame** and **Edward Lambert** at the Mayo Clinic, using electron-microscopy of freeze-fractured neuromuscular junctions.[12] The active zone particles were close enough to be spanned by two arms of an immune globulin (IgG) molecule, suggesting that these effects might be the result of antibodies cross-linking adjacent active zone particles.

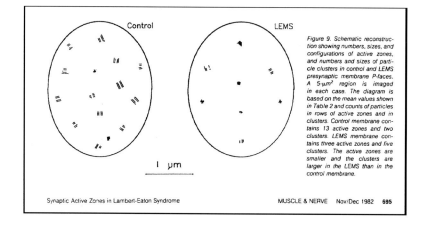

Figure 9. Schematic reconstruction showing numbers, sizes, and configurations of active zones, and numbers and sizes of particle clusters in control and LEMS presynaptic membrane P-faces. A 5-μm² region is imaged in each case. The diagram is based on the mean values shown in Table 2 and counts of particles in rows of active zones and in clusters. Control membrane contains 13 active zones and two clusters. LEMS membrane contains three active zones and five clusters. The active zones are smaller and the clusters are larger in the LEMS than in the control membrane.

Synaptic Active Zones in Lambert-Eaton Syndrome   MUSCLE & NERVE   Nov/Dec 1982   **695**

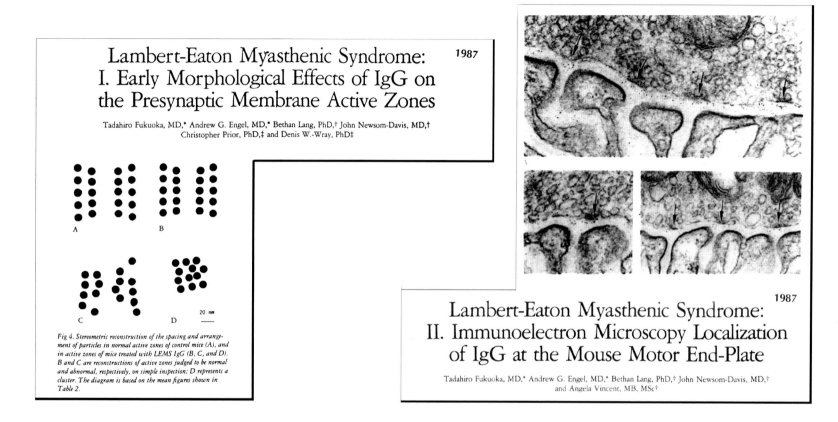

Lambert-Eaton Myasthenic Syndrome: 1987
I. Early Morphological Effects of IgG on the Presynaptic Membrane Active Zones

Tadahiro Fukuoka, MD,* Andrew G. Engel, MD,* Bethan Lang, PhD,† John Newsom-Davis, MD,†
Christopher Prior, PhD,‡ and Denis W.-Wray, PhD‡

A

B

C

D

20 nm

Fig 4. Stereometric reconstruction of the spacing and arrangement of particles in normal active zones of control mice (A), and in active zones of mice treated with LEMS IgG (B, C, and D). B and C are reconstructions of active zones judged to be normal and abnormal, respectively, on simple inspection; D represents a cluster. The diagram is based on the mean figures shown in Table 2.

Lambert-Eaton Myasthenic Syndrome: 1987
II. Immunoelectron Microscopy Localization of IgG at the Mouse Motor End-Plate

Tadahiro Fukuoka, MD,* Andrew G. Engel, MD,* Bethan Lang, PhD,† John Newsom-Davis, MD,†
and Angela Vincent, MB, MSc†

The two leading laboratories investigating LEMS at that time, one at the Mayo Clinic in Rochester, Minnesota, and the other at the Royal Free Hospital in London, England, collaborated in 1987 on two important papers. The first[13] by **Tadahiro Fukuoka, Andrew Engel, Bethan Lang, John Newsom-Davis, Christopher Prior,** and **Dennis Wray** showed that inoculation of serum IgG from LEMS patients into mice for several days produced similar disruption and clustering of active zone particles in the treated mice, indicating that "passive transfer" of antibody from LEMS patients could reproduce some of the features of the disease. In the second paper,[14] **Fukuoka, Engel, Lang, Newsom-Davis,** and **Vincent** showed that ferritin particles attached to LEMS IgG could be localized by sensitive "immuno-electron microscopy" to the active zones of mouse motor nerve endings, demonstrating directly that LEMS antibody interacted with a target at the presynaptic active zones. None of the treated mice became weak, but rodents have a "safety factor" of neuromuscular transmission and rarely demonstrate weakness, even in experimental autoimmune myasthenia gravis.

The results of these ultrastructural studies were confirmed by physiological experiments in 1987. **Lang, Newsom-Davis, C. Peers, Prior,** and **Wray**, studying the effect of various calcium concentrations upon miniature end-plate potential amplitude and frequency in phrenic nerve-diaphragm preparations, suggested that LEMS IgG produced a 30-40% reduction in the number of functional presynaptic voltage-gated calcium channels.[15]

Mirroring the progress in myasthenia whereby "gifts of nature" were used to develop radioimmune antibody assays, two toxins from cone shells and one from spider venom have been found which bind to various subsets of calcium channels. **E. Sher** and associates in 1989, were the first to report that antibodies against N-type voltage-gated calcium channels could be detected in 90% of sera from patients with LEMS but also in a large percentage of lung carcinoma patients without LEMS and even in some controls.[16] Similar findings among these groups of patients have recently been reported for antibodies against P/Q voltage-gated calcium channels. Furthermore, each type of calcium channel has several subunits with which LEMS antibodies apparently bind preferentially, so that the eventual significance of these assays cannot be predicted at this time.

References for Chapter 6, Part A: Lambert-Eaton Myasthenic Syndrome (1951-1989)

1. Anderson HJ, Churchill-Davidson HC, Richardson AT: Bronchial neoplasm with myasthenia, prolonged apnoea after administration of succinylcholine. *Lancet* 2:1291-1293, 1953.

2. Henson RA, Russell DS, Wilkinson M: Carcinomatous neuropathy and myopathy, a clinical and pathological study. *Brain* 77:82-121, 1954.

3. Heathfield KWG, Williams JRB: Peripheral neuropathy and myopathy associated with bronchogenic carcinoma. *Brain* 77:122-137, 1954.

4. Lambert EH, Eaton LM, Rooke ED: Defect of neuromuscular conduction associated with malignant neoplasms. *Amer J Physiol* 187:612-613, 1956.

5. Eaton LM, Lambert EH: Electromyography and electric stimulation of nerves in diseases of motor unit. Observations on myasthenic syndrome associated with malignant tumors. *J Amer Med Assn* 163:1117-1124, 1957.

6. Lambert EH, Rooke ED, Eaton LM, Hodgson CH: Myasthenic syndrome occasionally associated with bronchial neoplasm: Neurophysiologic studies. Section IV, Chapter 4, pp. 362-410, in *Myasthenia Gravis, The Second International Symposium Proceedings* (HR Viets, ed.), CC Thomas, Springfield, Illinois, 1961.

7. Elmqvist D, Lambert EH: Detailed analysis of neuromuscular transmission in a patient with the myasthenic syndrome sometimes associated with broncho-genic carcinoma. *Mayo Clinic Proceedings* 43:689-713, 1968.

8. Lindstrom JM, Lambert EH: Content of acetylcholine receptor and antibodies bound to receptor in myasthenia gravis, experimental autoimmune myasthenia gravis, and Eaton-Lambert syndrome. *Neurology* 28:130-138, 1978.

9. Gutmann L, Crosby TW, Takamori M, Martin JD: The Lambert-Eaton syndrome and autoimmune disorders. *Amer J Med* 53:354-356, 1972.

10. Denys EH, Dau PC, Lindstrom JM: Neuromuscular transmission before and after plasmapheresis in myasthenia gravis and the myasthenic syndrome. Chapter 23, pp. 248-257 in *Plasmapheresis and the Immunology of Myasthenia Gravis* (PC Dau, ed.), Houghton Mifflin, Boston, Massachusetts, 1979.

11. Lang B, Newsom-Davis J, Wray D, Vincent A, Murray N: Autoimmune aetiology for myasthenic (Eaton-Lambert) syndrome. *Lancet* 2:224-226, 1981.

12. Fukunaga H, Engel AG, Osame M, Lambert EH: Paucity and disorganization of presynaptic membrane active zones in the Lambert-Eaton myasthenic syndrome. *Muscle & Nerve* 5:686-697, 1982.

13. Fukuoka T, Engel AG, Lang B, Newsom-Davis J, Prior C, Wray D: Lambert-Eaton myasthenic syndrome: I. Early morphological effects of IgG on the presynaptic membrane active zones. *Ann Neurol* 22:193-199, 1987.

14. Fukuoka T, Engel AG, Lang B, Newsom-Davis J, Vincent A: Lambert-Eaton myasthenic syndrome: II. Immunoelectron microscopy localization of IgG at the mouse motor endplate. *Ann Neurol* 22:200-221, 1987.

15. Lang B, Newsom-Davis J, Peers C, Prior C, Wray DW: The effect of myasthenic syndrome antibody on presynaptic calcium channels in the mouse. *J Physiol London* 390:257-270, 1987.

16. Sher E, Canal N, Piccolo G, Gotti C, Scoppetta C, Evoli A, Clementi F: Specificity of calcium channel autoantibodies in Lambert-Eaton myasthenic syndrome. *Lancet* 2:640-643, 1989.

Congenital Myasthenic Syndromes, 1937-1990

Children who develop myasthenia have always been of special interest, ever since the first case—that of a previously healthy 2¾-year-old boy who died suddenly after a month's illness—was described in 1898 by **Max Mailhouse**, a neurologist at the Vanderbilt Clinic in New York City.[17]

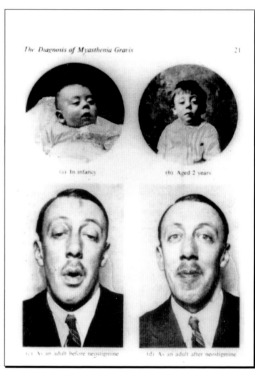

The child above, who appeared in Byrom Bramwell's 1892 Atlas of Clinical Medicine as "remittent oph-thalmoplegia of uncertain aetiology, attributed to syphilis," was pictured in Simpson's classic 1960 "autoimmune hypothesis" paper as "almost certainly a myasthenic child."

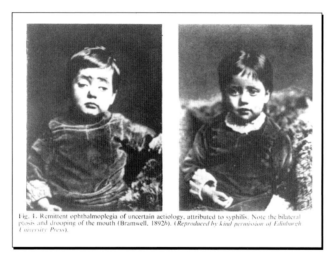

Fig. 1. Remittent ophthalmoplegia of uncertain aetiology, attributed to syphilis. Note the bilateral ptosis and drooping of the mouth (Bramwell, 1892). (*Reproduced by kind permission of Edinburgh University Press*).

From Raymond Greene: *Myasthenia Gravis, A Book*, Fig. 1, p. 21, William Heinemann Medical Books, LTD., London, 1969.

A special situation seemed to apply when the myasthenia occurred at birth and was therefore "congenital and perma-nent," as in this series of photographs of the same patient over time.[18]

M yasthenia that occurred in more than one child in a family was of particular interest, and was called "familial myasthenia." **Henry Hart** of Philadelphia, Pennsylvania, described two sisters in 1927 in whom myasthenia was recognized at ages 9 and 14 when they began to have menstrual periods.[19] In 1937 **Harold Rothbart** of Detroit, Michigan, reported four boys in one family who were affected with myasthenia before the age of two.[20] Two of the brothers are pictured on the left, below.

In 1949 **Paul Levin** of Dallas, Texas, described the onset of myasthenia at birth in two siblings,[21] one of whom is pictured below (center). Levin emphasized the "perfect symmetry" of the muscular weakness and the stability of the course. He differentiated this condition from the transient neonatal myasthenia which occurs in about 12% of infants born to mothers with autoimmune myasthenia and which is thought to result from antibodies crossing the placenta.

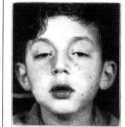
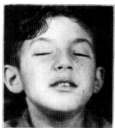
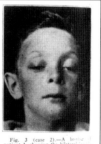

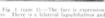
Fig. 1 (case 1).—The face is expressionless. There is a bilateral lagophthalmos and drooping of the mouth.

Fig. 2 (case 1).—Bilateral facial weakness shown when the patient is smiling.

Fig. 3 (case 2).—A brother of patient 1, showing the bilateral lagophthalmos.

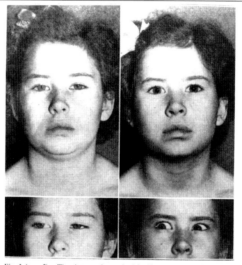

Fig. 3 (case 2).—The photographs on the left side were made before, and those on the right after, the injection of 1.5 mg. of neostigmine methylsulfate with 0.6 mg. of atropine sulfate. The lower pictures show the patient exerting maximal lateral gaze to the right. Minimal ptosis and limitation of ocular movements were seen before the injection, whereas afterward there were retraction of the upper lids, especially on lateral gaze, and an increase in range of ocular rotation. The ptosis and ocular paresis are symmetric.

TABLE 4
INFANTILE CASES OF MYASTHENIA GRAVIS*

Author	Sex of those affected	No. of normal sibs
Ramsay Hunt (1916)	F	2
Kawaichi and Ito (1942)	M	0
Yahr and Davis (1944)	F	2
Bowman (1948)	M	2
Wyllie et al. (1951)	F	1
Mackay (1951)	F	4
Walker (1953)	F	?
Macrae (1954)	M	3
Heinzen and Baasch (1955)	M	?
Teng and Osserman (1956)	3 M; 5 F	?
Millichap and Dodge (1960)	3 M; 2 F	?
Wiesendanger and Baasch (1962)	2 M	?
Oosterhuis (1964)	1 M; 2 F	?
Wolf et al. (1966)	1 M; 1 F	?
Present author (non-familial cases)	1 M; 3 F	7
Familial cases from Table 3	27 M; 9 F	11 +

* Those with onset at 2 years or under; excluding transitory neonatal myasthenia.

By 1972 **Sarah Bundey** in London, England, could compile 97 cases of familial or congenital "myasthenia gravis" in the medical literature (see Table 3 on the right), 41 of which presented before the age of 2 years.[22] (see Table 4, left).

A genetic study of infantile and juvenile myasthenia gravis

TABLE 3
FAMILIAL CASES OF MYASTHENIA GRAVIS*

Reference	Age of onset (yr.)	Affected individuals	Unaffected sibs (no.)
Sibs only affected: age of onset under 2 years:			
Rothbart (1937)	< 2	4 Bro.	2
Eaton (1947)	Infancy	2 Bro.	?
Levin (1949)	< 1	Bro. and Si.	0
Bornstein (1953)			
Kott and Bornstein (1969)	< 3 months	3 Bro. 1 Si.	1
Macrae (1954)	< 1	Bro. and Si.	4
Biemond and Trotsenburg (1955)	15/12	Dizygous male twins	?
Teng and Osserman, 1956	Birth	Bro. and Si.	?
Walsh and Hoyt (1959)	< 2	4 Bro.	2
Millichap and Dodge (1960)	Birth; birth; 1	Bro. and Si.	?
Warot and Delahousse (1964)	< 2	2 Bro.	0
Simpson (1964)	< 2	2 Si.	2
Herrmann (1966)	1 + 3	Bro. and Si.	0
Fessard et al. (1968)	6/12 and 8/12	Si. and Bro.	1
Gath et al. (1970)	Birth	Bro. and Si.	?
Present study	6/12 and 18/12	2 Bro.	0
Sibs only affected: age of onset after 2 years:			
Marinesco (1908)	21 + 31	2 Si.	?
Hart (1927)	9 + 14	2 Si.	?
Riley and Frocht (1943)	11 + 14	2 Si.	6
Mancusi-Ungaro (1945)	28 + 18	2 Si.	?
Teng and Osserman (1956)	?	Bro. and Si.	?
Goulon et al. (1960)	15 + 21	2 Si.	?
Greenberg (1964)	19 + 40	2 Si.?	?
Simpson (1964)	42 + ?	2 Si.	?
Celesia (1965)	6/12 + 8	Si. and Bro.	?
Herrmann (1966)	33 + 36	2 Bro.	1
Namba and Grob (1971)	29 + 39	2 Si.*	4
Present study	18 + 24	2 Si.	1
Other relatives affected:			
Noyes (1930)	?, 55 + 60	Fa. Son and Da.	
Bowman (1948)	3 + 4	1st cousins (M and F)	
Teng and Osserman (1956)	Childh.; 7	1st cousins (F and ?)	
	Birth; birth; 1	Bro. & Si. 1st cousin (M)	
Foldes and McNall (1960)	? + 2	Mo. and Son	
	17; 39 + 27	Mo. + 2 Da.	
Millichap and Dodge (1960)	?	Female child and 2 cousins	
Simpson (1964)	21 + 27	cousins (M and F)	
Haralanov and Kutchoukov (1966)	46 + 18	Fa. and Da.	
Herrmann (1966)	26 + 8	Fa. and Son	
	30's + 67	Sister and half-bros. Da.	
	55 + 71	2nd cousins (M and F)	
	77 + 51	1st cousins (2 F)	
Warrier and Pillai (1967)	16 + 12	Bro. and Si.	
	Birth; 2/12; 3	(nephews of above: parents are cousins	
Present study	10 + 4	Mo. and Son	

* Monozygotic twins are not included in this Table, nor are familial cases reported by Oppenheim (1898) and Hokkanen (1969a) which are not fully documented.
† These four affected sisters also had hyperthyroidism.

The difference between these cases of congenital or familial myasthenia and other cases of myasthenia gravis could not be recognized until the specific autoimmune nature of most myasthenia was discovered in the 1970's. However, congenital cases did not respond to thymectomy or immunosuppression, and never had elevated titers of acetylcholine receptor antibody in their sera. They were thus more likely to be of genetic than of autoimmune etiology.

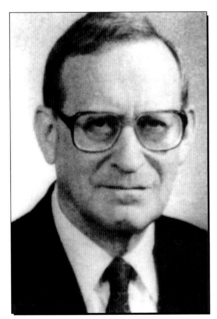

Andrew Engel

Once this distinction was made, several specific congenital myasthenic syndromes were characterized, especially at the Mayo Clinic under the leadership of **Andrew Engel**, who studied muscle biopsies from patients with these disorders by quantitative electron microscopy and cytochemistry, along with **Edward Lambert**, who used microelectrodes to analyze *in vitro* the electrophysiology of the same biopsies.

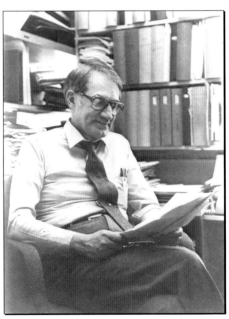

Edward Lambert

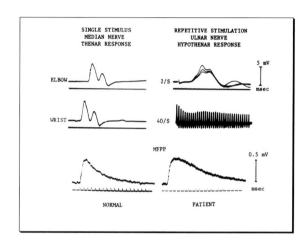

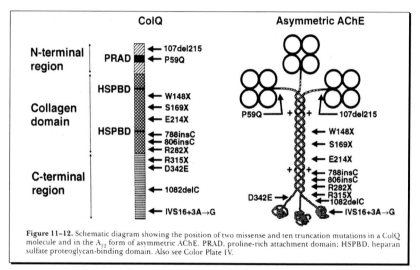

Figure 11–12. Schematic diagram showing the position of two missense and ten truncation mutations in a ColQ molecule and in the A$_{12}$ form of asymmetric AChE. PRAD, proline-rich attachment domain; HSPBD, heparan sulfate proteoglycan-binding domain. Also see Color Plate IV.

Reprinted with permission from *Myasthenia Gravis and Myasthenic Disorders* (AG Engel, ed.), Oxford University Press, New York, 1999, p. 271.

The first of these conditions to be described in detail by the Mayo group was "**Congenital Endplate Acetylcholinesterase Deficiency**" in a 16-year-old Hindu boy with lifelong symptoms of generalized weakness unresponsive to anticholinesterase medications.[23] A repetitive response to a single nerve stimulus and prolonged miniature endplate potential duration were present (see above on left). Biochemical studies indicated total absence of the endplate-specific asymmetric form of acetylcholinesterase. Since that 1977 paper, several more patients with this particular type of disorder have been described, and genetic studies have found various mutations in the three strands (ColQ) of the collagen-like tail of the endplate asymmetric acetylcholinesterase (diagram above on right[24]).

A ttention was called in 1975 to a potentially fatal yet treatable condition named "Familial Infantile Myasthenia Gravis" by **John P. Conomy, Morris Levinsohn,** and **Avroy Fanaroff**[25] in Cleveland, Ohio, although it may have been described first in 1960 as a case of "Myasthenia gravis in the newborn" by **Melvin Greer,** and **Marilyn Schotland**[26] from Columbia-Presbyterian Medical Center in New York (photo below). It is characterized by recurrent apnea or episodic respiratory depression during the first two years of life, treatable by anticholinesterase medications. These attacks may eventually improve if the patient survives exacerbations caused by infections or fevers.

**FAMILIAL INFANTILE
MYASTHENIA GRAVIS: A
CAUSE OF SUDDEN DEATH
IN YOUNG CHILDREN**

JOHN P. CONOMY, M.D.
MORRIS LEVINSOHN, M.D.
and
AVROY FANAROFF, M.D.
Cleveland, Ohio

From the Divisions of Neurology, Pediatric Neurology,
and the Department of Pediatrics, Case Western-Reserve
University Medical School, and University Hospitals of
Cleveland.

———

Reprinted from
THE JOURNAL OF PEDIATRICS
St. Louis

Vol. 87, No. 3, pp. 428-430, September, 1975
(Copyright © 1975 by The C. V. Mosby Company)
(Printed in the U.S.A.)

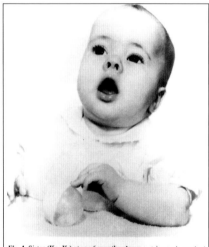

Fig. 1. Sister (Ka. K.) at age 6 months. Asymmetric ptosis, peaked lips, and habitually opened mouth are apparent. There is no atrophy of the face or other visible musculature.

**Session on Neuromuscular
Diseases I
Afternoon Meeting
Thursday, April 26, 1979**

2:30 P.M.—4:30 P.M.
Ballroom A, B, C

Chairman: Andrew G. Engle, Rochester, Minnesota
Secretary: Richard S. A. Tindall, Dallas

NMD 2—2:45

A Congenital, Familial Myasthenic Syndrome Caused by
a Presynaptic Defect of Transmitter Resynthesis or
Mobilization

ZWI H. HART, Detroit, K. SAHASHI, E. H. LAMBERT, and
A. G. ENGEL, Rochester, Minnesota, and J. M. LINDSTROM,
San Diego

A boy now age 18 (propositus) and his sister, now 5, had fluctuating ptosis since birth, feeding difficulty during infancy, easy fatigability on exertion, and episodic apnea following crying, vomiting, or febrile illnesses. Symptoms responded to prostigmine but not to prednisone, and improved with age. Three other siblings (myasthenic symptoms noted in two) died suddenly in infancy. The parents and two older sibs are asymptomatic. No circulating antibody to acetylcholine receptor (AChR) was found in any family member. Electromyography of the propositus showed a decremental response at 2-Hz stimulation after exercise, but not in the resting state. His external intercostal muscle contained a normal amount of AChR and no antibodies to AChR by radioimmunoassay and by quantitative immunoelectronmicroscopy. Morphometry of endplates revealed increased numbers of synaptic vesicles. Postsynaptic regions were normal. In rested muscle the miniature endplate potential (mepp) amplitude, the quantum content (m) of the endplate potential (epp) (at 1 Hz) and the probability of release and the number of immediately releasable quanta were normal. During 10-Hz stimulation for a few minutes, the epp amplitude decreased abnormally due to an abnormal decrease of the mepp amplitude and of m. The findings are consistent with a presynaptic defect of acetylcholine re-synthesis or mobilization.

The Mayo group reported in a 1979 abstract[27] (on the right) that the electrophysiological findings in this condition resembled normal muscle poisoned by hemicholinium, an inhibitor of choline uptake, and later small synaptic vesicles were seen on electron microscopy.[28] Recent studies have established that several different mutations of choline acetyltransferase, the enzyme which synthesizes acetylcholine, can cause the congenital myasthenic syndrome with episodic apnea (CMS-EA).[32]

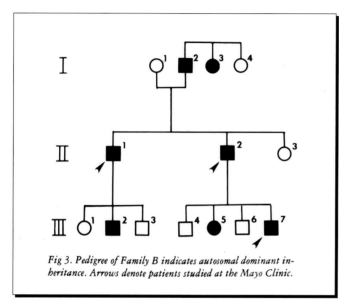

Fig 3. *Pedigree of Family B indicates autosomal dominant inheritance. Arrows denote patients studied at the Mayo Clinic.*

Another congenital myasthenic syndrome was described by **Engel, Lambert** and colleagues in 1982[29] based upon five familial cases in two families and one sporadic case. All had repetitive compound muscle action potentials to a single nerve stimulus in all muscles and markedly prolonged endplate potentials and miniature endplate potentials, unaffected by anticholinesterase medications, similar to the patients with acetylcholinesterase deficiency. However, the cause of this syndrome was found to be a prolonged open time of the acetylcholine-induced ion channel, which produced not only the above electrophysiological findings but allowed excessive calcium influx to produce an endplate myopathy. Subsequent molecular genetic studies of these "**Slow Channel Syndromes**" have demonstrated numerous dominant mutations in different parts of acetylcholine receptor subunits, most of them associated with the ion channel portions of the molecules resulting in an increased affinity for acetylcholine.[24]

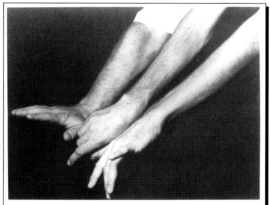

Fig 4. *Patient 5 attempting to extend his wrists and fingers as shown by examiner (with sleeve).*

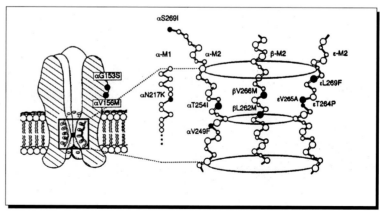

Reprinted with permission from *Myasthenia Gravis and Myasthenic Disorders* (AG Engel, ed.), Oxford University Press, New York, 1999, p. 276.

Accumulating evidence about these various congenital myasthenic syndromes has allowed them to be grouped into defects of presynaptic, synaptic and post-synaptic proteins. Most post-synaptic congenital myasthenic syndromes are associated with a kinetic abnormality or decreased expression of the acetylcholine receptor. Besides the dominant "slow channel syndromes" (see page 89), recessive "fast channel syndromes" have also been described—first in 1990[31]—in which there is decreased affinity for acetylcholine. Mutations of the collagenic tail subunit of the endplate species of acetylcholinesterase (see page 87) are examples of synaptic defects. Presynaptic syndromes include the choline acetyltransferase mutations producing episodic apnea (see page 88) as well as a congenital myasthenic syndrome resembling LEMS, first described in 1987.[30]

EACH OF THESE SYNDROMES, when thoroughly studied, has provided unique information about the importance of the multiple steps required for effective communication between nerve and muscle. It is possible that such "experiments of nature" may eventually contribute to a complete understanding of the marvel of neuromuscular transmission.

References for Chapter 6, Part B: Congenital Myasthenic Syndromes (1937-1990)

17. Mailhouse M: A case of myasthenia pseudo-paralytica gravis (Jolly) or asthenic pulbar paralysis (Strumpell). *Boston Medical & Surgical J* 138:439-441, 1898.

18. Greene R: *Myasthenia Gravis.* Heinemann, London, p. 21, 1969.

19. Hart HH: Myasthenia gravis with ophthalmoplegia and constitutional anomalies in sisters. *Arch Neurol Psychiat* 18:439-442, 1927.

20. Rothbart HB: Myasthenia gravis in children, its familial incidence. *J Amer Med Assn* 108:715-717, 1937.

21. Levin PM: Congenital myasthenia in siblings. *Arch Neurol Psychiat* 62:745-758, 1949.

22. Bundey S: A genetic study of infantile and juvenile myasthenia gravis. *J Neurol Neurosurg Psychiat* 35:41-51, 1972.

23. Engel AG, Lambert EH, Gomez M: A new myasthenic syndrome with end-plate acetylcholinesterase deficiency, small nerve terminals and reduced acetylcholine release. *Ann Neurol* 1:315-330, 1977.

24. Engel AG, Ohno K, Sine SM: Chapter 11, Congenital myasthenic syndromes, pp. 251-297 in *Myasthenia Gravis and Myasthenic Disorder*s. (AG Engel, ed.), New York, Oxford University Press, 1999.

25. Conomy JP, Levinsohn M, Fanaroff A: Familial infantile myasthenia gravis: A cause of sudden death in young children. *J Pediatrics* 87:428-430, 1975.

26. Greer M, Schotland M: Myasthenia gravis in the newborn. *Pediatrics* 26:101-108, 1960.

27. Hart ZH, Sahashi K, Lambert EH, Engel AG, Lindstrom JM: A congenital, familial, myasthenia syndrome caused by a presynaptic defect of transmitter resynthesis or mobilization. *Neurology* 29:556-557, 1979 (abstract).

28. Mora M, Lambert EH, Engel AG: Synaptic vesicle abnormality in familial infantile myasthenia. *Neurology* 37:206-214, 1987.

29. Engel AG, Lambert EH, Mulder DM, Torres CF, Sahashi K, Bertorini TE, Whitaker JN: A newly recognized congenital myasthenic syndrome attributed to a prolonged open time on the acetylcholine-induced ion channel. *Ann Neurol* 11:553-569, 1982.

30. Bady B, Chauplannaz G, Carrier H: Congenital Lambert-Eaton myasthenia syndrome. *J Neurol Neurosurg Psychiat* 50:476-478, 1987.

31. Engel AG, Walls TJ, Nagel A, Uchitel O: New recognized congenital myasthenic syndromes: I. Congenital paucity of synaptic vesicles and reduced quantal release, II. High-conductance fast-channel syndrome, III. Abnormal acetylcholine receptor (AChR) interaction with acetylcholine, IV. AchR deficiency and short channel-open time. *Progress in Brain Research* 84:125-137, 1990.

32. Ohno K, Tsujino A, Brengman JM, Harper CM, Bajzer Z, Udd B, Beyring R, Robb S, Kirkham FJ, Engel AG: Choline acetyltransferase mutations cause myasthenic syndrome associated with episode apnea in humans. *Proc Natl Acad Sci USA* 98:2017-2011, 2001.

Conclusion

The preceding six chapters have put into updated narrative form the six posters that were presented at the *Ninth International Conference on Myasthenia Gravis and Related Disorders* in Santa Monica, California, in 1997. As such, they include only those highlights of the history of myasthenia gravis that could be fitted on a poster. Each of the foregoing chapters should be viewed as an introduction to topics that could – and hopefully will – be treated in greater historical detail in the future.

Many important aspects of this subject have been left out completely. These include most of the non-specific treatments presently used to alleviate MG—pyridostigmine (Mestinon), prednisone, immunosuppressive medications and intravenous immunoglobulin (IVIG). David Grob's recent graph (on right) is instructive in this regard. The graph would suggest that although confirmation by electrical (repetitive nerve stimulation, 1941) and pharmacological (edrophonium [Tensilon], 1953) tests contributed to increased recognition, the prevalence of MG increased over the past century mainly because general respiratory support and antibiotics improved the survival of patients with MG. The modern era of diagnosis by serum acetylcholine receptor antibody (1975) and treatment with steroids (1966) and plasma exchange (1975) has produced relatively little change in the curves shown graphically.

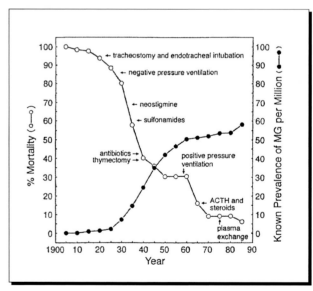

—from **David Grob**, "Natural History of Myasthenia Gravis," in *Myasthenia Gravis and Myasthenic Disorders* (AG Engel, ed.), New York, Oxford University Press, 1999, Fig. 6-1, p. 132, with permission.

The fascinating interactions that have played a crucial role in understanding the pathogenesis of myasthenia gravis need to be studied in any future MG history. An authoritative glimpse of these was given in 1990 by one of the leading investigators of the diseases of the neuromuscular junction.[1] After discussing a "first theme" – the latent period between a basic science observation and its clinical application – **Andrew Engel** then described the flow of influence from one investigator to the next in his own particular field of the neuromuscular junction (NMJ):

The second theme pertains to the manner in which basic science skills are transmitted from one investigator or laboratory to another. The transmission is by personal guidance of one investigator by another. For example, the application of in vitro microelectrode studies to the human intercostal muscles in Lund in the 1960's would not have come about without Stephen Thesleff's tutelage with Bernard Katz. The physiological defect in MG would not have been described by Elmqvist and co-workers without Thesleff's guidance. The introduction of microelectrode methods to the Mayo Clinic and the subsequent description of the physiological defect in the Lambert-Eaton syndrome by Elmqvist and Lambert in 1968 would not have come about without a visit by Dan Elmqvist to the Mayo Clinic that year. My own interest in the structure and function of the NMJ might not have been kindled had it not been for my association with Ed Lambert during that time.

Hopefully, others alive today who have made important contributions to our knowledge of myasthenia gravis will follow Dr. Engel's example and soon describe the important interactions that made their discoveries possible.

1. Thesleff S, Heilbronn E, Molenaar PC, Engel AG: Future prospects of cholinergic research on neuromuscular transmission. Chapter 19 in *Progress in Brain Research* 84, p.174, 1990.

GLOSSARY

ACETYLCHOLINE
A simple organic molecule made up of acetic acid and choline, which is liberated as a neurotransmitter by vertebrate motoneurons as well as by preganglionic autonomic neurons. It is broken down by the enzyme cholinesterase.

ACETYLCHOLINE RECEPTOR
A large molecule in the postsynaptic muscle membrane which combines with acetylcholine, causing a transformation of the shape of the molecule such that ions may pass through a pore in the molecule and excite the muscle.

ACETYLCHOLINE-RECEPTOR ANTIBODY TITER
An assay for antibodies in serum that bind to solubilized acetylcholine receptor molecules.

ACETYLCHOLINESTERASE
An enzyme that breaks acetylcholine into choline and acetic acid.

ACETYLCHOLINE SYNTHESIS
The production of acetylcholine from acetate and choline.

ACTION POTENTIAL
The electrical impulse of a single nerve or muscle fiber.

ACTIVE ZONE
A region on the presynaptic membrane at which synaptic vesicles are released into the synaptic cleft.

ALKALOID
An organic nitrogen-containing substance obtained from plants and used in certain drugs.

ALL-OR-NOTHING RESPONSE
A response to a stimulus that occurs only as a full-sized impulse; otherwise, there is no response. Contrasted with a graded response.

ALPHA-BUNGAROTOXIN
Toxin from the snake venom of the Formosan krait, *Bungarus multicinctus*, which binds to acetylcholine receptors with high affinity.

ANATOMICAL
Connected with anatomy, the study of the structure of animals and plants.

ANTERIOR MEDIASTINUM
The space in the body between the lungs, in front of the heart and great vessels, in which the thymus is located.

ANTIBODY
An immunoglobulin with a specialized combining site that reacts specifically with an antigen. (See "immunoglobulin")

ANTICHOLINESTERASES
Cholinesterase inhibitors, such as the drugs neostigmine (Prostigmin), edrophonium (Tensilon), and pyridostigmine bromide (Mestinon), which prevent the breakdown of acetylcholine and thereby allows the action of acetylcholine to be prolonged.

ANTIDOTE
A remedy to counteract a poison.

ANTIGEN
Any substance that provokes the production of specific antibody or that interacts specifically with products of the immune response.

ANTIGEN-ANTIBODY REACTION
The interaction between a specific antibody and its antigen.

ARMAMENTARIUM
Literally, an arsenal; in medicine, the methods used to combat illness.

ASTHENIA
Bodily weakness; a lack or loss of bodily strength.

ATROPHY
A wasting away of a body tissue such as a muscle.

ATROPINE
A cholinergic blocking drug used to counteract the muscarinic effects of acetylcholine.

AUTOIMMUNE
Immunized against a body's own constituents.

AUTONOMIC NERVOUS SYSTEM
That part of the nervous system supplying viscera, blood vessels, smooth muscle, glands and the heart, consisting of two distinct divisions, parasympathetic and sympathetic.

AUTOPSY
An examination and dissection of a dead body to discover cause of death; also termed a "necropsy" or "postmortem".

AUTOTOXIN
Any toxin or poison produced inside the body.

AXON
A nerve fiber; the principal process of a neuron conducting impulses over relatively long distances.

AZATHIOPRINE
An immunosuppressive drug, brand name "Imuran".

BASIC SCIENCE	Systemized knowledge concerned with the discovery of unknown laws relating to particular facts; "pure" science as opposed to "applied" science, the latter concerned with application of discovered laws to the matters of everyday living.
BIOCHEMISTRY	The branch of chemistry that deals with plants and animals and their life processes.
BIOPSY	In medicine, the excision of a piece of living tissue for diagnostic examination, usually by microscopy.
BLOCKING	In medicine, the prevention of an expected action, such as the blocking antibody in myasthenia which prevents the binding of acetylcholine to the acetylcholine receptor, or the effect that a drug such as curare has on preventing acetylcholine from stimulating the acetylcholine receptor.
BONE-MARROW-DERIVED LYMPHOCYTES	White blood cells originating in the bone marrow and called B cells, as opposed to those processed in the thymus and called T cells.
BRAINSTEM	That part of the central nervous system between the cerebral cortex and the spinal cord, containing centers for breathing and swallowing as well as the origin of nerves to the face, jaw, tongue, throat and diaphragm; the "bulb".
BRONCHIAL NEOPLASM	A cancer of the bronchus, either of two main branches of the trachea or windpipe.
BULBAR	Pertaining to the "bulb" or brainstem, which is normal in myasthenia. Therefore, it is more appropriate to use the term "oropharyngeal" when describing myasthenic weakness of the areas innervated by the bulb.
CAPILLARY	Any of the tiny blood vessels connecting the arteries with the veins.
CARBACHOL	A synthetic chemical with many actions similar to acetylcholine.
CARCINOMATOUS	Having the nature of, or affected by, cancer.
CARDIOLOGY	The study of the heart, its functions and its diseases.
CELL BODY	In biology, the part of the cell containing the nucleus and

	protein-manufacturing apparatus, as distinguished from cell processes, such as the axon of a nerve cell (neuron).
CENTRAL NERVOUS SYSTEM	The brain and spinal cord, as distinguished from the peripheral nervous system which consists of nerve cells and fibers in the rest of the body.
CHEMORECEPTOR	A receptor adapted for excitation by chemical substances.
CHOLINE	The simple precursor and breakdown product of acetylcholine.
CHOLINERGIC NEURONS	Neurons that release acetylcholine as transmitter.
CHOLINERGIC RECEPTOR	Another name for a receptor that binds acetylcholine.
CHOLINESTERASE	An enzyme that breaks down choline-containing compounds; acetylcholinesterase specifically breaks acetylcholine down into choline and acetic acid.
CHOLINESTERASE INHIBITOR	Another term for an anticholinesterase.
CLINICAL	Pertaining to a clinic or the bedside, founded on actual observation and treatment of patients, as distinguished from theoretical or experimental.
COLLAGEN	The main supportive protein of skin, tendon, bone, cartilage, and connective tissue.
COMPLEMENT	A complex system of plasma protein factors and enzymes capable of binding to and being activated by a large number of antigen-antibody systems.
COMPETITIVE BLOCKING	The term used to describe the action of certain drugs such as curare, which competes with acetylcholine for the active site of the acetylcholine receptor. It is distinguished from blocking which occurs as a result of loss of the membrane potential. (See "depolarization blocking")
COMPOUND MUSCLE ACTION POTENTIAL	The electrical change which is recorded from the surface of an entire muscle which has been stimulated by its nerve; it is the summation of the individual action potentials of all the active muscle fibers in the muscle.

CONGENITAL MYASTHENIC SYNDROMES — Various forms of persistent myasthenic weakness which has been present since birth on the basis of genetic changes in the apparatus of neuromuscular transmission, as distinguished from autoimmune myasthenia.

CONTRAINDICATION — Any condition or disease which makes an indicated medication or treatment inadvisable.

CORTICOSTEROIDS — Compounds chemically resembling cholesterol which include or resemble substances made in the adrenal cortex such as cortisone and corticosterone, possessing life-maintaining properties in animals lacking the adrenal glands. Prednisone is a synthetic corticosteroid.

CRISIS — A term used to describe respiratory insufficiency in myasthenia caused by weakness of the muscles of the throat, intercostal muscles and/or diaphragm to such an extent that the patient is unable to breathe adequately and requires mechanical assistance.

CURARE — A drug extracted from South American plants that paralyzes nerve-muscle transmission by occupying acetylcholine receptor sites.

CYANOTIC — Characterized by blueness of the skin, usually caused by insufficient oxygenation of the blood.

CYCLOSPORINE — An immunosuppressive drug.

CYSTIC — Pertaining to any sac, normal or otherwise, especially one which contains a liquid or semisolid substance.

DECAMETHONIUM IODIDE — A muscle relaxant used in anesthesia which blocks the action of acetylcholine by depolarizing the muscle membrane potential.

DECREMENTAL RESPONSE — The typical diagnostic response of a myasthenic muscle to repetitive nerve stimulation, in which more and more muscle fibers fail to fire during the first few stimuli so that the muscle response becomes smaller and smaller. After about five responses, however, reparative mechanisms stabilize and even increase subsequent responses towards normal.

DEGENERATION — Deterioration, change from a higher to a lower or less functionally active form.

DELTOID MUSCLE — A specific large shoulder muscle.

DEPOLARIZATION — Reduction towards zero of the normal resting potential across a membrane.

DEPOLARIZATION BLOCKING — The term used to describe the action of certain drugs such as decamethonium in which the action of acetylcholine is prevented because the muscle membrane potential is reduced by the drug towards zero.

DIAPHRAGM MUSCLE — The musculomembranous partition that separates the abdomen from the thorax and is the primary muscle used in expanding the chest during breathing.

DIPLOPIA — The perception of two images of one object; double vision.

DYSARTHRIA — Difficulty articulating speech because of weakness of muscles, to be distinguished from dysphasia, which is trouble understanding or finding words.

DYSPHAGIA — Difficulty swallowing.

DYSPLASTIC — Marked by abnormality of development; deformed.

DYSPNEA — Shortness of breath, difficulty breathing.

EDROPHONIUM — A short-acting anticholinesterase which is given intravenously as a test for myasthenia gravis; brand name "Tensilon".

ELECTROMYOGRAPHY — The recording of changes in electrical potential of a muscle by insertion of a needle electrode into the muscle and observing the action potentials at rest and during voluntary contraction, as a means of detecting the location and nature of motor unit lesions.

ELECTRON MICROGRAPH — The photograph of an object through an electron microscope, which magnetically focuses a beam of electrons instead of a beam of light onto a fluorescent screen.

ENDOTHELIUM	The layer of simple squamous (scaly or plate-like) cells which lines the inner surface of blood vessels.
ENDPLATE	Postsynaptic area of vertebrate skeletal muscle fiber.
ENDPLATE POTENTIAL	A postsynaptic electric potential in the endplate region of a skeletal muscle fiber produced by acetylcholine liberated from presynaptic nerve terminals.
EPHEDRINE SULFATE	An early drug found useful in myasthenia gravis.
EPITHELIAL RETICULUM	A network of epithelial cells.
EPITHELIUM	Cellular tissue that covers surfaces, forms glands and lines most cavities of the body, consisting of one or several layers of cells with only little intercellular material.
ESERINE	Another name for physostigmine, an anticholinesterase.
EXACERBATION	Increase in the severity of any symptoms or disease.
EXCITATION	Process tending to produce electric impulses (action potentials).
EXTRACELLULAR	Outside of a cell or cells.
EXTRAOCULAR MUSCLES	The six muscles around each eyeball which normally move the two eyes in exact synchrony to provide a fused image.
EXTREMITY	A limb; arm (upper extremity) or leg (lower extremity).
FACILITATION	Greater effectiveness of synaptic transmission by successive pre-synaptic impulses, usually due to increased transmitter release.
FALSE TRANSMITTER	A biologically inactive substance stored in and released by synaptic vesicles instead of a true neurotransmitter such as acetylcholine.
FATIGUE	In myasthenia, the decreased ability of a muscle to function because of repetitive physical exertion, distinguished from the much more common general fatigue such as weariness, physical or mental exhaustion.

FERRITIN	An iron-containing protein which is used as a marker in electron microscopy.
FETUS	In man, the offspring in the womb from the end of the third month of pregnancy until birth, distinguished from the earlier embryo.
FIBRILLARY SPASMS	An old-fashioned term for sustained contraction of muscle fibers.
FLUORESCENCE	The property of producing light while being acted upon by radiant energy such as ultraviolet rays or X-rays.
FREEZE-FRACTURE	The technique of splitting frozen tissue tangentially along membrane planes, so that both the outside and inside surfaces of membranes can be visualized by electron microscopy.
FUNCTIONAL	Of or pertaining to the specialized, normal, or characteristic action of any part or organ, as opposed to the structural aspect of that part or organ.
GANGLION	Discrete collection of nerve cells.
GENERALISATA	The term Jolly recommended when "myasthenia gravis pseudoparalytica" was generalized to many muscles; generalized MG.
GERMINAL CENTER	The highly organized aggregation of lymphocytes and other cells that develops (usually in lymph nodes) in response to antigenic stimulation.
GLOBULIN	A class of proteins operationally classified as being insoluble in water (compared to albumin) but soluble in saline solutions. One of the purified globulin fractions, gamma globulin, contains the antibodies or immunoglobulins.
HEMOCHOLINIUM	A drug that interferes with acetylcholine synthesis by reducing or preventing the uptake by the nerve terminal or choline, which is needed for replenishment of transmitter in the terminals.
HYPERPLASIA	Increased cellularity, an abnormal increase in the number of normal cells in normal arrangement in a tissue.

HYPERPOLARIZATION	An increase in membrane potential from the resting value, tending to reduce excitability.
HYPERTHYROIDISM	Excessive functional activity of the thyroid gland, characterized by over-production and release of thyroid hormone, diffuse goiter, and infiltrative ophthalmopathy; called "Grave's Disease" in the English-speaking world and "Basedow's Disease" on the continent of Europe.
HYPOREFLEXIA	Decreased force of the tendon reflexes.
IMMUNE GLOBULIN (IG)	See immunoglobulin.
IMMUNITY	The protection of an organism against infectious agents or toxic antigens, afforded by a variety of predominantly specific factors.
IMMUNIZATION	The process of rendering a subject immune, as by an inoculation.
IMMUNO-ELECTRON MICROSCOPY	A very specialized procedure in which antibodies, bound to iron-containing ferritin, are localized by electron microscopy.
IMMUNOFLUORESCENCE	A method in which antibodies coupled to fluorescent molecules are employed as histochemical markers to identify or localize antigens or antibodies under the ultraviolet microscope.
IMMUNOGLOBULIN (IG)	A general term referring to all serum globulins that possess antibody activity.
IMMUNOHISTOCHEMISTRY	A term describing the study of immune mechanisms by histochemistry, the study of chemical substances in body tissues on a cellular scale.
IMMUNOLOGY	The branch of medicine dealing with the study of immunity to disease.
IMMUNOPEROXIDASE	Enzyme used as a histochemical marker from tracing antibodies as well as processes of neurons or spaces between cells.
IMMUNOSUPPRESSION	The non-specific diminution or elimination of immune responses by drug treatment or irradiation.

IMPULSE	Brief regenerative all-or-nothing electrical potential that propagates along an axon or muscle fiber; also called an "action potential".
INCOMPETENT CELLS	Cells which are unable to perform their required functions.
INDIGENOUS	Born, growing or produced naturally in a region or country; native.
INTERCOSTAL MUSCLES	Short muscles between the ribs, used in breathing.
INTRACELLULAR	Situated or occurring within a cell or cells.
INTRAVENOUS IMMUNE GLOBULIN (IVIG)	Gamma globulin antibodies pooled from thousands of human donors, suspended in aqueous solution by recent techniques and administered by intravenous infusion as a temporary immunosuppressive.
INTUBATION	The insertion of a tube into the windpipe for the purpose of establishing an airway to expedite breathing by mechanical assistance.
ION	An electrically charged atom or group of atoms, caused by the loss or gain of one or more negative electrons.
IONTOPHORESIS	Transfer of ions by passing current through a micropipette, used for applying charged molecules with a high degree of temporal and spatial resolution. Also called "electrophoresis".
JUNCTIONAL	In this book, pertaining to the neuromuscular junction where the nerve terminal and the muscle endplate come together.
LABELLING	To attach a marker, such as radioactivity or ferritin, to a substance for the purpose of identifying the location of that substance in tissue or in a biochemical separation.
LEUKEMIC NEOPLASM	A tumor of white blood cells (called leukocytes) and of their precursors.
LIANA	Any luxuriantly growing woody tropical vine that roots in the ground and climbs around tree trunks.

LUPUS ERYTHEMATOSIS DISSEMINATUS	A systemic disease associated with visceral lesions and characterized by skin eruptions, prolonged fever and other constitutional symptoms, thought to be autoimmune. Also called systemic lupus erythematosis (SLE).
LYMPH NODE	Any of the many gland-like structures lying in groups along the course of the lymphatic system.
LYMPHOCYTE	A variety of white blood cell associated with chronic inflammation, divided into several subgroups of which the most prominent are bone-marrow-derived lymphocytes (B cells) and thymus-dervied lymphocytes (T cells).
LYMPHORRHAGE	An accumulation of lymphocytes, especially in muscle.
LYMPHOSARCOMA	A malignant neoplasm arising in lymphatic tissue from proliferation of atypical lymphocytes.
MACROMOLECULE	A large molecule.
MALIGNANT	Very harmful or dangerous, likely to cause death; not benign.
MASSETER MUSCLES	Jaw muscles used for chewing.
MEDULLA	The central part of an organ such as the adrenal or thymus, as contrasted with its cortex. Also used to describe the lower part of the brainstem or bulb.
MEMBRANE	The structure constituting the surface of cells.
MEMBRANE POTENTIAL	The electrical potential across the cell membrane.
MESTINON	The brand name for pyridostigmine bromide, an anti-cholinesterase.
METASTASIS	The transfer of disease from one organ or part to another not directly connected with it. Plural: metastases.
MICROELECTRODE	A fine conductor, either a glass tube filled with conducting salt solution and with a tip diameter on the order of a micron, or a metal wire coated with insulation except at the tip, used to measure electrical events inside single cells.
MINIATURE ENDPLATE POTENTIAL	A small depolarization at a neuromuscular synapse caused by spontaneous release of a single quantum of acetylcholine from the presynaptic terminal.
MOTONEURON (MOTOR NEURON)	A large neuron, with its cell body in the central nervous system, that innervates muscle fibers.
MYASTHENIA GRAVIS (MG)	A neurological disease associated with fluctuating weakness and fatigue of skeletal muscles without sensory changes.
MYOID CELL	A cell found in the thymus resembling striated muscle.
MYONEURAL	Pertaining to both nerve and muscle; neuromuscular.
MYOPATHY	Any disease of muscle.
NECROTIC	Pertaining to the death or decay of a cell or group of cells which is in contact with living tissue.
NEONATAL MYASTHENIA	Transitory weakness in an infant born to a myasthenic mother.
NEOPLASM	Any new and abnormal growth of tissue, such as a tumor.
NEOSTIGMINE BROMIDE	An anticholinesterase drug, brand name "Prostigmin".
NERVE FIBER	Any of the thread-like elements making up a nerve; an axon.
NERVE TERMINAL	The enlarged ending of a nerve, specialized to contain packets of neurotransmitter to be released upon receipt of a nerve impulse.
NEURASTHENIA	Formerly, weakness or exhaustion of the nervous system as from excessive expenditure of energy; nervous prostration. Now, a type of neurosis, usually the result of emotional conflicts, characterized by a wide variety of symptoms, including fatigue, depression, worry, and often localized pains without apparent objective causes.
NEUROLOGY	The branch of medicine dealing with the nervous system, its structure and its diseases.

NEUROMUSCULAR	Pertaining to nerves and muscles.
NEUROMUSCULAR JUNCTION	The site at which the motor nerve terminal and the muscle endplate come together; myoneural junction.
NEUROMUSCULAR TRANSMISSION	The passage of the signal of the nerve impulse from the nerve terminal by release of acetylcholine into the synaptic cleft, and stimulation by acetylcholine of the acetylcholine receptors on the muscle endplate, with the subsequent opening of ion channels in the receptors to create an action potential along the muscle membrane.
NEURON (NERVE CELL)	The biological unit of the nervous system.
NEUROTOXIN	A substance that is poisonous or destructive to nerve tissue.
NEUROTRANSMITTER	(See transmitter.)
NOMARSKI INTERFERENCE CONTRAST MICROSCOPY	In contrast to the two-dimensional image of ordinary bright-field microscopy, interference contrast microscopy uses a beam of polarized light split into two beams, one of which courses through the object (suspended in solution) while the other doesn't, and when the beams are recombined this results in a "three-dimensional" or "shadow-cast" image.
NUCLEUS	(A thing or part forming the center, around which other parts or groups are collected.) The spheroid body within a cell containing the genetic material. Also, a group of nerve cells in the central nervous system.
OCULAR MYASTHENIA	Myasthenic weakness confined to the ocular muscles, resulting in fluctuating double vision and drooping eyelid(s).
PALSY	Paralysis, loss or impairment of motor function.
PARANEOPLASTIC	Abnormal function, especially of the nervous system, caused by the remote presence of a tumor, usually a cancer, presumed to be the result of cross-reaction of immune responses against the tumor with components of the nervous system.
PARESIS	Incomplete paralysis.

PASSIVE TRANSFER	In experimental medicine, the reproduction of features of an antibody-mediated disease in one animal by simple intravenous injection of antibodies from another animal.
PATHOGENESIS	The production or development of a disease.
PATHOLOGY	That branch of medicine that studies the essential nature of disease, especially of the structural and functional changes in tissues and organs of the body that cause or are caused by disease.
PERIPHERAL NEUROPATHY	Any disease or disorder of the peripheral nervous system.
PHARMACOLOGY	The science that deals with the study of drugs.
PHRENIC NERVE-DIAPHRAGM PREPARATION	An experimental preparation consisting of the phrenic nerve of an animal attached to the diaphragm it innervates, often used to study neuromuscular transmission.
PHYSICK	An archaic term for a medicine or remedy, or in general for the art or science of healing.
PHYSIOLOGICAL	Pertaining to physiology, the science which studies the functions of the living organism and its parts.
PHYSOSTIGMINE	An alkaloid that reversibly inhibits the effects of acetylcholinesterase; also called eserine.
PITUITARY GLAND	A small oval endocrine gland attached by a stalk to the base of the brain that secretes several hormones which influence other endocrine glands.
PLASMAPHERESIS	Literally, the drawing off of plasma, the non-cellular component of unclotted blood. In practice, the plasma is replaced by salt solutions and albumin. This isn't literally "plasma exchange" (plasma for plasma). However, "plasmapheresis" and "plasma exchange" are used synonymously.
POLIOMYELITIS	Inflammation of the gray matter of the spinal cord, especially infantile paralysis. Also called "polio".
POLYCLINIC	A hospital or clinic for the treatment of all kinds of diseases and injuries. Compare to policlinic, the outpatient department of a city hospital.

POST-MORTEM — An examination made after death; autopsy, necropsy.

POSTSYNAPTIC MEMBRANE — The muscle cell membrane immediately related to the synapse formed by presynaptic fibers.

POST-TETANIC EXHAUSTION — The decremental decline in the size of an evoked compound muscle action potential which sometimes occurs in myasthenia a few minutes after the muscle has been exercised.

POTENTIAL — In electricity, the relative voltage at a point in an electric circuit or field as referred to some other point in the same circuit or field.

PREDNISONE — A synthetic corticosteroid often used to treat myasthenia gravis.

PRESYNAPTIC FIBERS — The terminal branches of nerve fibers that end at synapses.

PROGNOSIS — A prediction of the probable course of a disease and the chances of recovery.

PROSTIGMIN — Brand name for neostigmine bromide, an anticholinesterase.

PROTEIN — Any of a class of nitrogenous substances consisting of a complex union of amino acids and comprising the chief constituents of cells.

PROTOPLASM — A semifluid, viscous, translucid colloid with water as the continuous phase, the essential matter of all living animal and plant cells.

PROXIMAL MUSCLES — Those muscles situated nearest the center of the body or the point of attachment of a limb, as opposed to distal muscles.

PSEUDOPARALYTICA — False paralysis, the term Jolly used to modify "myasthenia gravis," implying fluctuating loss of muscular power with normal reflexes.

PSYCHIATRY — The branch of medicine concerned with the study and treatment of disorders of the mind.

PTOSIS — Droopiness of an eyelid or both eyelids, caused by muscle weakness, which usually fluctuates in myasthenia.

PULMONARY — Pertaining to the lungs.

PUPILLARY SPHINCTER — The smooth muscles in the iris of the eye which contract and dilate the opening at the center of the iris which is called the pupil.

PYRIDOSTIGMINE BROMIDE — Anticholinesterase drug commonly used in myasthenia; generic name for brand name, "Mestinon".

QUANTAL RELEASE — Release of multimolecular packets (quanta) of transmitter by the presynaptic nerve terminal, occurring either spontaneously or evoked by a nerve impulse.

RADIOACTIVE — Giving off radiant energy in the form of particles or rays, as alpha, beta and gamma rays, by the disintegration of atomic nuclei.

RADIOGRAPHS — A picture produced on a sensitized film or plate by rays other than light rays, especially by X-rays; an X-ray picture.

RADIOIMMUNO-PRECIPITATION ASSAY — The method used to measure blocking and binding antibodies in sera, in which radioactive alpha-bungarotoxin is bound to the acetylcholine sites of the acetylcholine receptor either before (binding) or after (blocking) the serum antibody is attached to the receptor; the complex is then precipitated by an anti-antibody and the radioactivity counted.

RECEPTOR — A molecule in the cell membrane that combines with a specific chemical substance.

REMISSION — A clinical condition in which a patient who has had myasthenia no longer takes medication and has no symptoms. Lack of symptoms while taking medication is called a drug-dependent remission.

REPETITIVE NERVE STIMULATION — A diagnostic test for myasthenia in which a nerve is stimulated electrically supra-maximally at a repetitive frequency while each response of the whole muscle innervated by that nerve is recorded.

RESPIRATION	The function of breathing; the act by which air is drawn in and expelled from the lungs.
RESTING POTENTIAL	The steady electrical potential across a biological membrane in the quiescent state.
RETICULOENDOTHELIAL SYSTEM	A group of cells with both endothelial and reticular attributes, particularly macrophages, in the spleen, lymph nodes, bone marrow, concerned with blood cell formation and destruction.
RHEUMATOID ARTHRITIS	A chronic disease characterized by inflammation, stiffness and often deformity of the joints of the body, thought to be autoimmune.
ROENTGENOTHERAPY	Therapeutic use of roentgen rays (X-rays or gamma rays).
SAFETY FACTOR	Regarding neuromuscular transmission, the excess amount by which the endplate potential exceeds the threshold for muscle action potential propagation.
SARCOIDOSIS	A chronic disease of unknown cause marked by characteristic lesions in the skin, lymph nodes, salivary glands, eyes, lungs and bones.
SCHWANN CELL	The supporting cell which produces each segment of peripheral myelin, a fatty insulating substance wrapped around each myelinated nerve fiber.
SECTION	A very thin slice of matter used for microscopic study.
SENSORY NERVES	Nerves concerned with the reception and transmission of sense impressions, such as touch, pain and position sense. Special sensory nerves transmit information about vision, hearing, taste, and smell.
SERUM	In the clotting of blood, the clear liquid which separates from the clot and blood cells (plural: sera).
SIGN	In medicine, any objective evidence of disease, distinguished from a symptom.
SMOKED DRUM	Part of a kymograph, an instrument containing a rotating drum covered with a thin layer of soot on which a needle records variations such as muscular contractions or pulse.
STERNAL	Pertaining to the sternum or breast bone, a plate of bone forming the middle of the anterior wall of the chest.
STRIATED MUSCLE	Muscle, the fibers of which are divided by transverse bands into striations. Such muscles are under voluntary control. Also formerly called "striped" muscle.
SUBCUTANEOUS	Situated or introduced beneath the skin.
SUPRAMAXIMAL STIMULATION	An amount of stimulation greater than needed to produce a maximum response.
SUPRARENAL	Situated above the kidney, specifically designating an adrenal gland.
SYMPTOM	Usually a subjective complaint offered by a patient, contrasted with an objective sign of disease. However, dictionaries define "symptom" as "any condition accompanying a disease and serving as an aid in diagnosis."
SYNAPSE	Specialized site at which neurons communicate by chemical or electrical transmission with other neurons or with effector organs such as muscle.
SYNAPTIC CLEFT	The narrow space between the membranes of the presynaptic and postsynaptic cells at a chemical synapse across which transmitter must diffuse.
SYNAPTIC VESICLES	Small membrane-bound sacs in presynaptic nerve terminals that contain neurotransmitters such as acetylcholine.
TAGGED	Labelled; attached with a marker, such as radioactivity or ferritin, for the purpose of identification in the body or during a biochemical separation.
TENDON REFLEXES	Simple reflex actions produced by tapping a tendon, the pathway for which involves a single synapse between a sensory nerve and a motoneuron. They are often called "deep" tendon reflexes to distinguish them from superficial skin reflexes.

TENSILON

The brand name for edrophonium chloride, a rapid-acting anticholinesterase used as an intravenous diagnostic test for myasthenia.

TETANUS

In physiology, the continuous tonic spasm, or steady contraction without distinct twitching, of a muscle undergoing a rapidly repeated stimulus.

THRESHOLD

Critical value of membrane potential depolarization at which an electrical impulse is initiated.

THYMECTOMY

Surgical removal of the thymus gland.

THYMOMA

Tumor of the thymus gland consisting of lymphocytes and epithelial cells.

THYMUS GLAND

A variable organ lying in the neck and between the breast bone and the heart, which processes immature lymphocytes to become thymus-derived T cells in the circulation.

THYROIDITIS

Inflammation of the thyroid gland.

THYROTOXICOSIS

Manifestations of excess thyroid hormone at the level of peripheral tissues; hormone could be ingested as well as overproduced.

TOURNIQUET

Any device for compressing a blood vessel to stop bleeding or to prevent the access of blood to some part of the body.

TRANSMITTER

Chemical substance liberated by a presynaptic nerve terminal that causes an effect on the membrane of the postsynaptic cell, usually an increase in permeability to one or more ions.

TREATISE

A formal systematic essay or book on some subject.

TUMOR

A mass of new tissue growing independently of its surrounding structures and having no physiologic function; a neoplasm.

TWITCH

In physiology, a brief, sudden, quick contraction of a muscle, contrasted with a tetanic contraction.

ULTRAVIOLET MICROSCOPE

A microscope with quartz lenses used chiefly for photography with ultraviolet light.

VESICLES

In neuromuscular transmission, small sacs containing neurotransmitter seen in the nerve terminal under the microscope.

VESTIGIAL

In biology, rudimentary, atrophied, degenerated, undeveloped.

VITAL CAPACITY

The number of milliliters of air a person can forcibly expire after a full inspiration.

VOLTAGE-GATED CALCIUM CHANNELS (VGCC)

Ion channels in membranes of nerve cells, and of cells in some lung tumors derived embryologically from neural tissue, which allow calcium ions to cross the cell membrane when a depolarizing voltage gradient is applied.

WHITE BLOOD CELLS

Leukocytes; colorless nucleated cells in the blood which include lymphocytes, macrophages and polymorphonuclear leukocytes, contrasted with the red blood cells which carry hemoglobulin and have no nucleus.

List of Illustrations

63	photomicrograph & tables	from *Neurology*, 1972, vol. 22, pp. 77-76, with permission from Lippincott Williams & Wilkins.
64	photo of snake on left	from Steven Novom, M.D., with permission.
64	figure of diaphragms on right	from *Nature* (London), 1967, vol. 215, pp. 1177-1178, with permission.
65	photo of Jean-Pierre Changeux	from *Cold Spring Harbor Symposia on Quantitative Biology*, 1976, vol. XL, p. xii.
65	drawing of Torpedo	from *Essays on the History of Italian Neurology* (Luigi Belloni, ed.), 1961, Studi E Testi 6, Instituto di Storia Della Medicino, Universita degli studi, Milano.
66	photo of Douglas Fambrough	from *Cold Spring Harbor Symposia on Quantitative Biology*, 1976, vol. XL, p. xiii.
66	figure of autoradiographs	from *Science*, 1972, vol. 176, pp. 189-190, with permission of the American Association for the Advancement of Science.
67	photo of Daniel Drachman	from Daniel B. Drachman, M.D., with permission.
67	figure of autoradiographs	from *Science*, 1973, vol. 182, pp. 193-195, with permission of the American Association for the Advancement of Science.
68	photo of Jon Lindstrom	from Myasthenia Gravis Foundation of California, with permission.
68	photo of Jim Patrick & Raftery	from *Cold Spring Harbor Symposia on Quantitative Biology*, 1976, vol. XL, p. xiii.
69	model of receptor	from *Cold Spring Harbor Symposia on Quantitative Biology*, 1983, vol. XLVII, pp. 89-99.
69	photos of rabbits & tracings	from *Science*, 1973, vol. 180, pp. 871-872, with permission of the American Association for the Advancement of Science.
70	photo of Lindstrom, Lennon & Seybold	from Myasthenia Gravis Foundation of California, with permission.
70	figure of graph	from *Neurology*, 1976, vol. 26, pp. 1054-1059, with permission of Lippincott Williams & Wilkins.
71	photo of panelists	Source unknown.
71	figure of graph	from *Lancet*, 1976, vol. 2, pp. 1373-1376, reprinted with permission from Elsevier Science.
72	photo of mice	from *New England J Medicine*, 1977, vol. 296, pp. 125-130, with permission of the Massachusetts Medical Society.

CHAPTER 6

76	article title page on left	from *Lancet*, 1953, vol. 2, pp. 1291-1293, reprinted with permission from Elsevier Science.
76	journal title page on right	from *Brain*, 1954, vol. 77, part I, with permission of Oxford University Press.
77	photo of Edward Lambert	from Mayo Clinic Yearbook, with permission of the Mayo Foundation.
77	abstract	from *American J Physiology*, 1956, vol. 187, pp. 612-613, with permission of the American Physiological Society.
77	photo of Lee Eaton	from Mayo Clinic Yearbook, with permission of the Mayo Foundation.
78	article title and summary on left	from *J American Medical Assoc*, vol. 163, p. 1117, copyrighted 1953 by the American Medical Association, with permission.

CONCLUSIONS

Index

A

acetylcholine, 39, 55, 56, 57, 58, 59, 61
acetylcholine receptor, 65, 66, 67, 68, 69, 70, 71, 75, 89
acetylcholine resynthesis or packaging, 88
acetylcholinesterase, 66, 69, 87, 88, 89
active zones, 79, 80, 81
alkaloid, 29, 30
Almon, Richard, 70
alpha-bungarotoxin, 64, 65, 66, 70
Amazon River, 33
American Journal of Cancer, 18
American Physiological Society, 77
Anderson, H.J., 76
Andrew, Clifford, 70
anterior mediastinum, 15
antibody, 49, 68, 69, 70, 71, 72, 75, 80, 82, 86, 92
anti-cholinesterase, 55, 57
anti-curare, 55
antigen-antibody reaction, 50
apnea, 76
Appel, Stanley, 70
Archiv fur Psychiatrie und Nervenkrankheiten, 2
asthenic bulbar palsy, 8, 9
atropine, 37
Australia, 52, 70
autoimmunity, 49, 55, 68, 72, 75, 79, 86, 92
autopsy, 2, 10, 16, 17, 20
autoradiographs, 66, 67
azathioprine, 92

B

Bady, B., 90
Baltimore, 45, 48, 66
Belgium, 26
Bell, Elexious T., 17, 18
Bender, Adam, 70
Bennett, A.E., 56
Berlin, 6, 8
Berliner Klinische Wochenschrift, 6
Bernard, Claude, 33, 34
biopsy, 26, 61, 86

Blalock, Alfred, 45, 46
Boerhaave, Herman, 24
Boothby, Walter M., 32
Boston, 48
Brain, 48, 76
brainstem, 1, 2
Bramwell, Byrom, 84
British Medical Journal, 41
bronchogenic carcinoma, 76
bulb, 1
bulbar palsies, paralysis, 1, 2, 5, 7, 10
Bulbarparalyse ohne anatomischen Befund, 8
Bundey, Sarah, 85
Bungarus multicinctus, 64
Buzzard, E. Farquhar, 20

C

Calabar bean, 36, 37
calabash-curare, 33
calcium, 79, 82, 89
calcium channel, 82
carcinomatous neuropathy, 76, 77
Carmichael, Arnold, 48
Carnegie Institution, 66
Cedars-Sinai Medical Center, 23
central nervous system, 1, 15, 16
Chang, Chuan-Chiung, 64
Changeux, Jean-Pierre, 65
Charcot, Jean Martin, *v,* 1, 15
Charite Hospital, 6
Chen, K.K., 31
Chester Beatty Research Institute, 52
Chiu, T.H., 64
choline, 58, 59
cholinergic receptor, 65
cholinesterase, 55, 57
Chondodendron, 33
Christison, Robert, 36
Chui, Luis, 26
Churchill-Davidson, H.C., 57, 76
circulating factor, 50, 92
Clagett, O. Theron, 46, 47
Cleveland, 88

Coërs, C., 26, 59
Columbia-Presbyterian Medical Center, 88
Columbia University, 31, 50, 51
competitive block, 58
complement, 50
congenital endplate acetylcholine deficiency, 87
congenital myasthenic syndromes, 75, 84, 85, 86, 89, 90
Conomy, John P., 88
Coutts, Stephen M., 3
curare, 29, 33, 34, 35, 38, 56, 64, 76
cyclophosphamide, 92
cyclosporine, 92

D

Dale, Sir Henry, 39
Dallas, 85
Daniels, Mathew, 70
Dau, Peter, 79
De Anima Brutorum, 11
decamethonium, 57, 61, 76
Denys, Eric, 79
Desmedt, J.E., 26, 59
Detroit, 85
Deutsche Zeitschrift for Nervenheilkunde, 4
Dioscorides, 29
Drachman, Daniel, 67, 72
Drinker, Philip, 43
dual response, 57, 58
Duane, Drake, 70
Duchenne de Bologne, 1, 5
Duke University, 70
dysplastic, 26
dyspnea, 5

E

Eaton, Lee, 46, 47, 77, 78
Eaton-Lambert Syndrome, 78
Edgeworth, Harriet, 31
Edinburgh, 36, 38
electric eel, 64, 65, 68

M

ma huang, 30
Mailhouse, Max, 84
Marstellar, 12
Masland, Richard, 56
Massachusetts General Hospital, 5
materia medica, 29, 36
Mayer, Sigmund, 23
Mayo Clinic, 32, 46, 47, 48, 62, 70, 77, 79,
    80, 81, 86, 87, 88, 90, 93
Medical Research Council Fellowship, 48
Mestinon, 55, 92
methylene blue, 26
Michigan, 85
microelectrode, 60, 61, 79, 86, 93
microscope, electron, 26, 60, 62, 63, 80
microscope, light, 24, 25, 26
Miledi, R., 65
Miller, Jacques F.A.P., 52
miniature end-plate potentials, 61, 82, 87, 89
Minnesota, 17, 18, 32, 77
Molinoff, P., 65
Molnar, Karin I., 5
monograph, 8
morbid anatomy, 15, 24
Mount Sinai Hospital, 50, 51
mouse, 72, 81
muscle, 16, 20, 22, 24, 25, 34, 49, 50, 51,
    56, 61, 66, 67, 70, 75, 76
myasthenia, 6, 9
myasthenia gravis clinic, 5, 50
myasthenia gravis pseudoparalytica, 6, 7
myasthenic syndrome, 75, 76, 77, 78
myoid cells, 23, 24
myoidzellen, 23
myoneural junction, 24, 34, 55
myopathy, 76

N

Nagai, Nagayoshi, 30
Nashville, William, 45, 50

Nastuk, William, 50, 52
National Institutes of Health, 51, 70
National Hospital for Nervous Diseases, 48, 71, 79
National Taiwan University, 64
Nebraska, University of, 56
negative pressure chamber, 43
neonatal myasthenia, 85
neostigmine, 40, 58, 68, 69, 76
nerve terminal, 55, 60
Neurologisches Centralblatt, 16
neuromuscular junction, 24, 39, 62, 63, 64,
    65, 72, 80, 93
neuromuscular transmission, 51, 57, 58, 60, 67, 90
neurotoxin, 64
New End Hospital, 48
New York City, 23, 50, 59, 84, 88
Newsom Davis, John, 71, 79, 81, 82
Nomarski interference contrast microscope, 25
Norris, Edgar Hughes, 18

O

Ohio, 88
Oosterhuis, Hans, 10, 51
Opechankanough, Chief, 12
Oppenheim, Herman, 6, 8, 16, 56
ordeal bean, 36
Osame, Mitsuhiro, 80
Osserman, Kermit, 50, 55
Osler, William, 9
Oxford University, 11

P

Pal, J., 35
Pappenheimer, Alvin, 23
paresis, 2, 5
Paris, 1, 65
passive transfer, 72, 81
pathology, 16, 17, 18
patient, 44, 45
Patrick, Jim, 68, 69

Peers, C., 82
Pennsylvania, 56, 85
pernicious anemia, 79
Peters, D.K., 71
pharmacology, 35
Philadelphia, 8, 85
photograph, 8
photomicrograph, 25, 26
Physostigma venenosum, 29, 36
physostigmine, 35, 37, 38, 39, 40, 55
Pinching, A.J., 71
plasma exchange, 71
plasmapheresis, 71, 79
Plescia, Otto, 50
poliomyelitis, 43
Pordage, 11
Post-activation exhaustion, 59
postsynaptic, 55, 56, 61, 63, 66
Potter, L.T., 65
Prague, 23
prednisone, 92
presynaptic, 55, 59, 61, 63, 75, 79, 80, 82
Principles and Practice of Medicine, 9
Prior, Christopher, 81, 82
Pritchard, E.A. Blake, 41
progressive bulbar palsy, 1, 2, 15
Prostigmin, 40, 41, 55, 68
ptosis, 2, 3, 5, 12, 50, 76
pupillary sphincter, 37
pyridostigmine, 55

Q

quantum, 61, 79
Quastel, D.M.J., 61
Queen Square, 48

R

rabbit, 68, 69
Raftery, M.A., 68
remission, 4, 5, 46

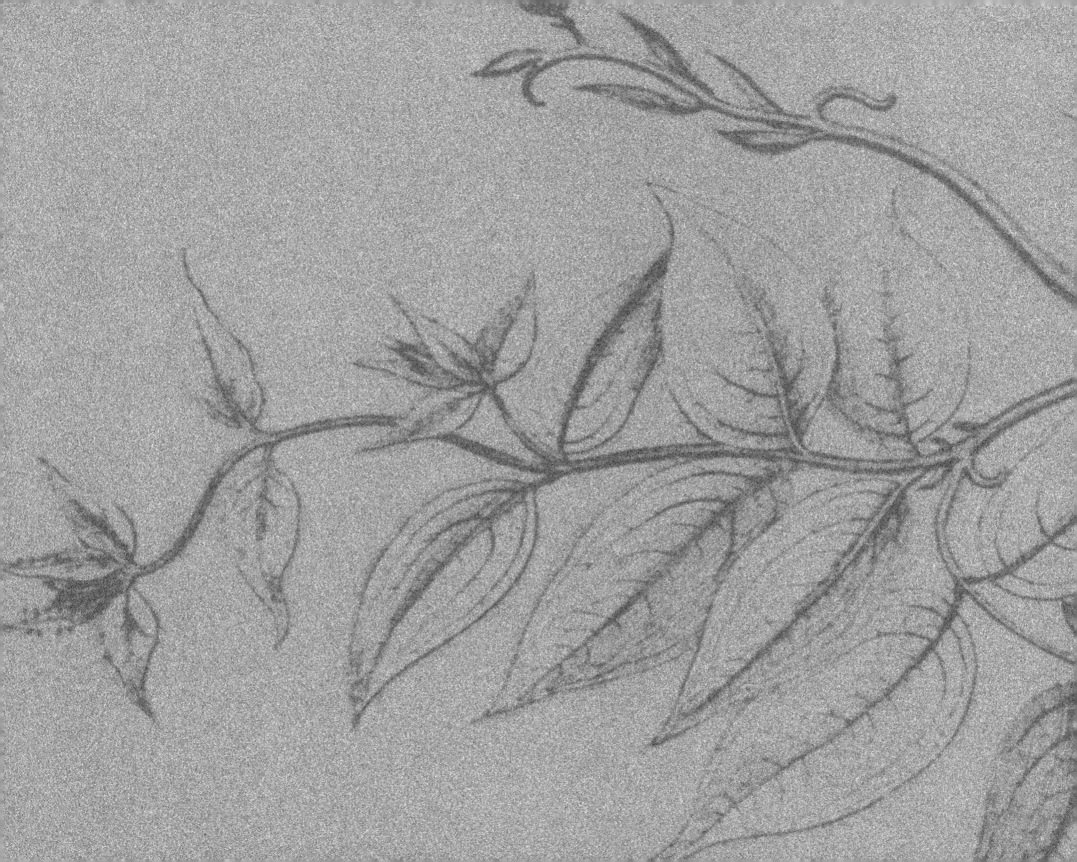